Disease and Medical Care

in the Mountain West

Wilbur S. Shepperson Series

in History and Humanities

Disease and Medical Care

in the Mountain West

Essays on Region, History, and Practice

E D I T E D   B Y

Martha L. Hildreth & Bruce T. Moran

University of Nevada Press / Reno, Las Vegas

Winner of the Wilbur S. Shepperson Humanities Book Award for 1997

This book is the recipient of the Wilbur S. Shepperson Humanities Book
Award, which is given annually in his memory by the Nevada Humanities
Committee and the University of Nevada Press. One of Nevada's most
distinguished historians, Wilbur S. Shepperson was a founding board
member and long-time supporter of both organizations.

Wilbur S. Shepperson Series in History and Humanities
Series Editor: Jerome E. Edwards

University of Nevada Press, Reno, Nevada 89557 USA
Copyright © 1998 by University of Nevada Press
All rights reserved
Manufactured in the United States of America
Design by Carrie Nelson House

Library of Congress Cataloging-in-Publication Data
Disease and medical care in the mountain West : essays on region, history,
and practice / edited by Martha L. Hildreth and Bruce T. Moran.
    p.   cm. — (Wilbur S. Shepperson series in history and humanities)
    Includes bibliographical references and index.
      ISBN 0-87417-304-3 (alk. paper)
      1. Medicine—West (U.S.)—History. I. Hildreth, Martha Lee.
    II. Moran, Bruce T. III. Series: Wilbur S. Shepperson series in history
    and humanities (Unnumbered)
      R154.5.W47D57 1997   97-26959
      610'.979—dc21   CIP

First Printing

07 06 05 04 03 02 01 00 99 98   5 4 3 2 1

Dedicated to students of the history of medicine in the Great Basin

CONTENTS

Foreword: *Todd Savitt*   ix

Acknowledgments   xi

Introduction: *Martha L. Hildreth & Bruce T. Moran*   xiii

1   The Significance of Regions in American Medical History   1
  Ronald L. Numbers

2   Steaming Saints: Mormons and the Thomsonian Movement in Nineteenth-Century America   18
  Thomas J. Wolfe

3   Suicide in the Nevada Hinterlands: A Cultural Perspective   29
  Marie I. Boutté

4   White Father Medicine and the Blackfeet, 1855–1955: Native American Health and the Department of the Interior   43
  Diane D. Edwards

5   The Scientific Construction of New Diseases: Rocky Mountain Spotted Fever and AIDS as Comparative Case Studies   59
  Victoria A. Harden

6   "Many Have Died and Others Must": The Silicosis Epidemic in Western Hardrock Mining, 1900–1925   72
  Alan Derickson

7   Frontier Nursing: The Deaconess Experience in Montana, 1890–1960   82
  Pierce C. Mullen

8   Chinese Medicine on the "Gold Mountain": Tradition, Adaptation, and Change   95
  Paul D. Buell

Notes   111

Contributors   141

Index   143

ILLUSTRATIONS

John Wesley Powell's Map of the Physiographic Regions
of the United States   2

Daniel Drake, M.D.   5

Hydrographical Map of the Interior Valley of North America   6

Epidemiological Subregions of the Southern United States
before the Civil War   7

Cabins for Tuberculosis Patients, New Mexico   9

Medical Schools in the United States and Canada, and
Recommended Locations of Medical Schools, 1910   10

Logo of the University of Washington School of Medicine
Primary Care Teaching Program   12

The Mormon Culture Region   14

Logo of the *Rocky Mountain Medical Journal*   15

Advertisement for the *Pacific Medical Record*   16

Nevada Highway 50 Sign   33

Montana Blackfeet at agency headquarters, 1889   47

Housing at Blackfeet reservation, 1951   47

In the fall of 1993 I had the privilege of attending the conference in Reno, Nevada, graciously hosted by Martha Hildreth and Bruce Moran, from which the papers in this book derive. The diversity of those papers provided an excellent introduction to the medical history of a region about which I knew little but in which I had recently developed a keen interest. I, a New Yorker who had devoted most of my career to studying regional medical history in the American South, was about to spend a semester teaching the history of medicine to undergraduates, health professionals, and other interested parties in Missoula, Montana. The West had hardly figured in my lectures and reading assignments for my usual history of medicine courses. Geographically, I noted with dismay, those courses, other than briefly mentioning Rocky Mountain spotted fever and the decimation of Native Americans by disease as white settlers moved westward in the nineteenth century, barely ventured beyond the Great Plains. Yet in a few months I would be teaching people who lived beyond the Plains and who would expect to learn how their region connected with, influenced, and was influenced by the medical history of the rest of the country. It occurred to me that I knew very little about the medical history of the West, and particularly the mountain West.

How could I get a handle on that history and find a way to weave it into my teaching? The Reno conference came to the rescue by putting the mountain West into the larger context of American medical history and by forcing me to see aspects of that history from a new perspective. Topics such as hospitals, nursing, Thomsonianism, Native American/white American medical interactions, silicosis and other industrial diseases, Chinese medicine, and the recognition and definition of diseases after the discovery of germs, all familiar territory to me as a medical historian, took new twists and held different meanings when placed in a western setting. The conference papers also demonstrated the uniqueness of mountain western medical history. The physical setting—climate, topography, and distance—was, I discovered, a powerful force that greatly affected the way the region was settled and the way people used the land on which they lived and worked. These settlement and work patterns, in turn, influenced the kinds of diseases from which people suffered. The people, too, were different from many of those back East. By the time settlers from the United States entered the region, Native Americans and persons of Spanish, Mexican, French, and Canadian heritages were already interacting, trading diseases and health practices. Shortly after the arrival of large numbers of American citizens from the East in the mid-nineteenth century, Chinese immigrants added their distinctive medical presence to the mix. The Reno conference showed how these various combinations of land and people affected the medical history of the mountain West. I was thus able to view the region's continuity with general American medical history while at the same time recognizing its uniqueness. This idea of western continuity and uniqueness reminded me of what I had found in studying southern medical history: regional history is important.

Some of the people who presented their research at the conference and whose papers are contained in this volume live in the mountain West; others have conducted research on and written about this section of the country for years. All of them know regional and medical history well. They provide an inspiring, scholarly introduction to both. Western medical history is an area that, like the region itself, is just being discovered by historians. Those of us who want to explore the region and its medical history need to learn the lay of the land before we begin our work. The papers in *Disease and Medical Care in the Mountain West* offer a fine model of how to go about doing this.

Todd Savitt
Greenville, North Carolina

ACKNOWLEDGMENTS

The papers in this volume were first presented at a conference, "Place and Practice: Regional Medicine, Health, and Health Care in the Intermountain West," held at the University of Nevada, Reno, October 22 and 23, 1993. We are grateful to the Nevada Humanities Committee and the Great Basin History of Medicine Committee for their generous support of the conference. The editors would especially like to acknowledge Dr. Anton Sohn (Chair, Department of Pathology, University of Nevada School of Medicine) and Dr. Ronald L. Numbers (William Coleman Professor of the History of Science, University of Wisconsin-Madison) for their continued encouragement of this project.

This volume explores the relationship between regionalism, health, and health care within a distinct section of the western United States. Questions about regionalism and the history of medicine have been asked before, but none have yet focused on the area loosely defined as the mountain West—an area bounded by the Rocky Mountains, Sierra Nevada, and Cascade Mountains. Whether or not the mountain West can be treated as a distinct geographical and cultural region is, of course, open to debate. Regardless of the artificiality of specific boundaries, however, this region is defined by a distinct environment. The physical surroundings of rock, mountains, and desert can seem overwhelming in this exposed, arid landscape. To live here often means living in isolation, far from other communities. The sense of separation is reinforced by a physical peculiarity of that part of the mountain region known as the Great Basin (the area between the Wasatch Mountains and the Sierra Nevada). There, rivers flow inward rather than reaching toward other people and places.[1]

The region's environment has shaped its culture and economy in many ways. Nineteenth-century immigrants from the eastern United States found farming nearly impossible, and most did not stay long. Mormons were the exception, taking advantage of the very difficulties that discouraged others to create a culture separate from mainstream society and religion. Chinese immigrants also found a niche after satisfying the labor demands of the railroads and mines that had brought them to the place they named the "Gold Mountain." Those who have had the longest presence in the mountain West are, of course, Native Americans, whose persistence in the region in the face of white immigration has been often related to a landscape not valued by others but sacred to them. Each of these groups—Mormon, Chinese, and Native American—preserved its own distinct set of attitudes toward the body, disease, and medicine.

Mining, ranching, and, in the twentieth century, tourism form the economy of much of the mountain West. The occupations connected with these industries have created communities of transients. This is particularly true in much of Nevada and Montana, where immigration patterns have been described as "cumulative"; that is, characterized by waves of diverse, disconnected individuals. Urbanization has been historically slow in coming. Many towns, following industrial patterns of boom and bust, began as mostly male communities. These communities often lacked traditional structures of family life and were, when illness and injury occurred, unable to depend on the traditional caretaking skills of women. Again, the Mormons are the exception. In Utah, immigration took the form of colonization, as existing communities relocated en masse and created a permanent culture based on farming.[2] While patterns of immigration differ in the mountain West, there is one common pattern: human society there is everywhere dispersed; mines, ranches, farms, towns, and individuals are often spread over immense distances.

Vast spaces and widely dispersed communities make the mountain West difficult to define by standard regional models, which focus on local nodes of authority and social organization such as cities and states. Instead, this region, thanks to the presence of enormous parcels of federal land, sometimes finds its guardians and policy makers (appointed officials from the Bureau of Land Management, the Bureau of Indian Affairs, and the Department of Defense) residing in places so far distant as to invoke comparison to a mythical Oz. From the perspective of many who call the mountain region home, it is an area that has historically been ill served by a health care system defined by hospitals, urban regional centers, group practice, and specialists. These problems continue into the present. There are only five medical schools in all of Wyoming, Montana, Idaho, Nevada, Utah, and New Mexico. A chronic shortage of rural physicians continues to be a major health concern and guides the politics of medical education.

How can the concept of region inform the history of medicine? The history of medicine has often been portrayed as the story of dedicated researchers using science to unveil biology and overcome the challenge of disease. Scholarship over the last twenty years has fundamentally altered this view, however, by taking into account social and cultural factors.[3] What David Arnold notes in regard to cholera applies equally to all disease: "Like any other disease, [it] has in itself no meaning: it is only a micro-organism. It acquires meaning and significance from its human context, from the ways in which it infiltrates the lives of the people, from the reactions it provokes, and from the manner in which it gives expression to cultural and political values."[4] Thus, the way society collectively gives meaning to the experience of disease can be viewed as a matter of cultural construction. Region constitutes a context for exploring that meaning and may reveal distinct cultural responses to institutions and disease. The notion that our understanding of the meaning of disease and medical practice is culturally constructed applies also to our understanding of death, a experience where medical practice and cultural meaning meet most dramatically.

Yet, the notion that diseases are cultural constructions must be weighed against a biological reality in which disease exists quite outside human culture and history. As Victoria Harden argues in her essay in this collection, disease must be understood as a natural phenomenon that historians should approach empirically. Charles Rosenberg makes a similar point in his important earlier study, *Framing Disease:* aside from those diseases that obviously cry out for what Rosenberg terms "social constructionist" analysis (e.g., neurasthenia, alcoholism, and anorexia nervosa), most disease has a clear biopathological phenomenology. Thus, in the face of Arnold's insistence that disease considered apart from culture is "only a micro-organism," Rosenberg and Harden want to call attention to the fact that the microorganism—its pathology and etiology—is fundamental to the study of the history of medicine. Is this an impasse? Perhaps the very concept of region offers a way of bridging the division.

Thomas McKeown has suggested that biopathology—the process of disease—rests finally on the material conditions of the host population.[5] In his view, influences such as nutrition, poverty or affluence, and the conditions of labor are profound and perhaps even determinate sources of disease causation. Regional factors define the immediate circumstances under which these material conditions affect human life. Poverty will have different consequences in remote isolation than in densely inhabited urban neighborhoods. Nutrition too depends on local circumstances. In winter, rural Nevadans of all economic levels have difficulty obtaining fresh fruits and vegetables. Thus, region may be seen as sculpting the essential conditions of disease and as framing the social response.[6]

The essays presented in this volume suggest that regionalism, as a basis for medical history, cuts across social constructionist and empiricist points of view. Region provides an analytical framework for studying the interaction of physical environment and human society. In fact, this collection reveals that the mountain West is a composite of different environments: cultural, geographic, economic, religious, epidemiological, and so on. It may be premature to argue that the distinct physical context—the arid climate, human isolation, and ranching and mining–based economy—constitutes a medical region comparable to the American South. Nevertheless, the essays in this volume open a discussion of the distinct health and health care identities of the mountain West.

Ron Numbers notes that regionalism has attracted only sporadic interest from medical historians, a situation that he insists needs redress. While the Southeast has been intensely explored by historians such as John Harley Warner and Todd Savitt, other regions have as yet almost no medical history. In a way, region is a forgotten category of medical thought. As Numbers observes, antebellum doctors and their patients assumed that illness was directly related to climate and physical environment; different regions had different diseases. Since then, medical thinking has moved in the direction of scientific universalism—each case of a disease is thought to be essentially the same, regardless of the locale. However, it took some time for regional thinking to disappear altogether. Conscious of their isolation, physicians in the mountain West created their own regional organizations and publications. The *Rocky Mountain Medical Journal,* founded in the early part of this century by regional societies, assumed that the existence of common diseases in the area gave the journal a raison d'être.

Numbers provides many suggestions for exploring various meanings of regionalism within the mountain West. Some of his observations—the importance of cultural groups such as the Mormons, for example—are illustrated elsewhere in this collection. Other issues, such as the impact of health-seeking tuberculosis immigrants and the largely unknown effects of what Numbers refers to as "hierarchical regionalism" in public health, remain to be investigated. Alongside arguments tending to support the concept of place as a foundation for studying medicine in the mountain West, Numbers also takes note of the porous boundaries of the area and the need to be aware of the fact that regions may be "nodal" rather than "uniform" and may be cultural, and epidemiological, rather than rigidly physiographic.

Epidemiology, more than any other factor of medical history, underscores the importance of region. Two essays in this volume examine the role of place in the medical construction of disease.

Victoria Harden observes that scientists and the lay community often have different understandings of diseases. Offering Rocky Mountain spotted fever and AIDS as examples, she explains how even in the twentieth century diseases sometimes become associated with a specific region. Harden points out that even when the scientific understanding of a disease's etiology has erased the stamp of regional identity, the identification of a disease with a specific region may continue within the general culture. The public continues to think that Rocky Mountain spotted fever is linked to a specific geographical area even though the scientific community has altered its original assumptions about the disease's regional derivation. The same may also be true of AIDS, which was initially identified by the medical community as an urban disease. Harden asks us to reject a narrow causal connection between place and disease and to consider a "situational association." Disease, she argues, is situated at the juncture of biopathological factors, environment, and human behavior.

Harden further directs our attention to the common elements of an intellectual matrix (or thought collective) that scientists use to frame experiments and to produce data leading to medical understanding of pathological processes. Her emphasis is more on the collectivity than on the individual scholar and amounts to regionalism of a different sort—a professional regionalism bounded by both emotional and intellectual constraints, preferred ways of seeing and feeling that have much to do with the construction of facts and ideas.[7]

Alan Derickson finds a less ambiguous relationship between place and disease in his analysis of miners' silicosis. Derickson describes the transformation of miners' silicosis from an occupational disease to an epidemiological phenomenon as the result of rapid industrialization and the application of new technology to mining. Political and economic factors peculiar to the mountain region, Derickson argues, delayed recognition of pneumoconiosis as an epidemic and forced hardrock miners themselves, through the Western Federation of Miners, to agitate for environmental and technological changes in the mines. Measures aimed at reducing the cause of the disease, such as underground ventilation standards and wet methods of dust abatement, were of foremost concern. In this case, new technology (often imposed because of statutory mandate) helped to cure what earlier technology had helped to cause, and an epidemic returned to the level of an endemic occupational disease.

Occupation also plays a role in another health-related concern in the mountain West: suicide. Marie Boutté examines the cultural context of suicide in a remote area of eastern Nevada. As a medical anthropologist, Boutté is sensitive to the creation of specific cultural constructions of disease—or in this case of the cultural construction of life and death. Boutté's compelling picture of suicide in Ely leads us to examine the geographical, economic, and occupational factors of this construction. Cultural practices such as risk taking, self-reliance, and the boom-and-bust economy that characterize societies based on ranching and mining appear to have created a climate that justifies suicide for some individuals. Boutté's analysis also demonstrates the limitations of traditional epidemiological approaches that rely on purely statistical data. Extrapolations from the data to the human behaviors must be carefully derived; one must go beyond the apparent truth of statistics and take cultural values into account. Boutté suggests that similar studies of urban Nevada and other parts of the mountain West will be needed to determine how cultural elements relate to specific human behaviors.

Diane Edwards discusses the health needs of Native Americans at the end of the nineteenth and during the first half of the twentieth century. Her study reveals problems created by circumstances typical of the area: lack of local control, isolation from centers of power, and the paternalism of government agencies. In northern Montana a displaced government bureaucracy with conflicting goals proved, in many respects, disastrous to the well-being of the Blackfeet population. The primary goal of the early policy was to turn the Blackfeet into Christian farmers. Health care was made available at schools created for this purpose, thus linking medical practice with "civilizing motives." Although successes as well as failures marked the history of the Department of the Interior's Blackfeet Agency, in the final analysis the public image of the strong and proud Native American contrasted sharply with the reality of reservation misery, disease, and starvation. Edwards's study is more than a survey of bureaucratic breakdown. In large part she is also concerned with how regionalism, distance, and isolation govern public perception. Only when a few outsiders actually visited the Montana reservation did local officials and Washington bureaucrats begin to feel the pressure of an outraged public. Like Derickson, Edwards shows how the disease problems of individuals are often caught within larger structures imposed by outside forces (economic-mining, governmental/bureaucratic-reservation). It's easy to be overlooked in the West; out of sight, out of mind.

Pierce Mullen takes note of a similar mixture of spiritual and practical goals, in this case as an essential part of Montana's nursing history. The Deaconess movement in Montana, like other nursing programs, combined a system of craft apprenticeship with missionary zeal. The nurses' Methodist mission combined caring for the body with a concern for salvation and spirituality. The practical and spiritual traditions affected nursing instruction as hospital service conflicted with university education and the ideals of nursing professionals collided with the moral concerns of administrators of Methodist hospitals. Isolation and impermanence created further difficulties as hospitals struggled to find women to nurse in the wards and colleges struggled to find adequate resources to educate them.

The trail of Methodism intersects another important religion in the West, Mormonism. Thomas Wolfe examines the interaction between medicine and religion, focusing on the interesting relationship between Mormonism and Thomsonian medical ideology. Even after Thomsonianism had died out in most of the rest of the country, it remained powerful within Mormon communities. By drawing attention to the cultural, political, and rhetorical traditions within each movement, Wolfe helps to explain the affinity of one for the other. In this colonized region, Mormon society achieved a degree of independence that allowed lawmakers to legislate formally against allopathy and in favor of Thomsonian remedies.

For Chinese immigrants to the frontier West, the "Gold Mountain" was a land of opportunities. The absence of well-organized centers of medical authority allowed these immigrants to pursue their own medical and pharmaceutical practices. Paul Buell looks at what happened when traditional Chinese medicine was adapted to the new environment. Generally, Chinese practices adhered steadfastly to ancient custom; however, traditional precedents were also expanded and directed toward the cure of local illnesses. On occasion, Chinese practice reached outside the Chinese community and a centuries-old Chinese tradition of herbal remedies found its way into communities of very different ethnic backgrounds, adding to the health care alternatives available to regional residents.

The peculiar environment and cultures of the mountain West have created a distinctive medical marketplace and have affected the roles and responsibilities of caregivers. Although the essays in this volume suggest a range of topics and approaches, the history of medicine in the region—both in its general outline and in its specialized studies—remains largely unwritten. Potentially fruitful courses of inquiry abound. Attention should be directed to medicine among the Basques, a very important cultural group of Idaho, Nevada, and Montana. Research into the intersections of Native American and Euro-American medical practices will also contribute to a fuller understanding of the region and its inhabitants. In addition, diseases peculiar to the mountain West and the special significance of the region as a therapeutic locale (as noted by Numbers) are areas of research that beckon future scholars. The history of spas and sanatoria, as well as of general and specialized hospitals, is another potential avenue of research. Recently completed oral histories of Nevada physicians suggest that a fascinating story remains to be told concerning the history of small-town medical practice in isolated and transient communities throughout the region.[8]

With so much promise for future scholarship, the authors assembled here have secured a place as pioneers charting a new domain in American medical history.

Disease and Medical Care

in the Mountain West

1   The Significance of Regions in

American Medical History

RONALD L. NUMBERS

Just over a century ago, a young historian at the University of Wisconsin—Frederick Jackson Turner—wrote one of the most important essays in American historiography. Prosaically titled "Problems in American History," it appeared in 1892 in a most unlikely place, a Madison student newspaper. In this piece Turner announced his discovery of two important factors in the development of a unique American society: the ever-retreating frontier and the distinct sections created as new settlers occupied particular physiographic regions. Turner, who soon found scientific support for the latter idea in the geographical work of John Wesley Powell, devoted the rest of his career to developing and popularizing the notions of frontier and section. Before his retirement he had come to view the sections of the United States as being roughly comparable to the countries of Europe, each possessing a distinctive culture and together forming a "nation of sections."[1]

Turner's sectionalism flourished in an America enamored of environmentalist explanations and still under the sway of intense regional loyalties. But academic interest in regions waned as the federal government expanded its role at the expense of the individual states and new technological developments such as radio and television, automobiles and airplanes increasingly homogenized American culture. This was especially true of the period after World War II, when so-called consensus historians stressed national unity and common purpose over diversity and conflict. By the 1970s, however, regionalism was making a modest comeback, especially among social scientists. This new regional-

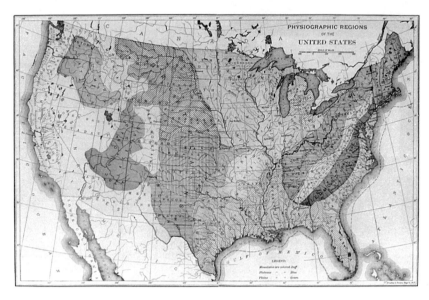

John Wesley Powell's map of the physiographic regions of the United States. From *The Physiography of the United States* (New York: American Book Company, 1896), 98–99.

ism focused more on culture than on climate. For example, in *Cultural Regions of the United States* (1975), Raymond D. Gastil largely ignored physical environments while emphasizing the cultural homogeneity within thirteen large areas. On the basis of cultural distinctives, he divided the mountain West into three regions: the Rocky Mountain, "dominated by ranching, mining, and irrigated oasis agriculture"; the Mormon, "the best-defined region in the nation"; and the interior Southwest, a culturally heterogeneous area unified in part by Roman Catholicism.[2]

The new American regionalists also derived inspiration from the *Annales* school in France, especially from Fernand Braudel, whose regional study *The Mediterranean and the Mediterranean World in the Age of Philip II* (translated into English in the early 1970s) transcends traditional national boundaries and religious divisions. Although widely cited, Braudel's work seems to have inspired few similar studies in the United States.[3]

One might expect regionalism to have benefited from the recent calls for attention to diversity in American society, but the advocates of diversity and multiculturalism have focused almost exclusively on race and gender, to the exclusion, for example, of region and religion; even class often receives scant attention. "Multiculturalists care little more about class as a fully elaborated identity . . . than they do about differences between religions, regions, and nations," laments the historian John Higham. "To its academic apostles, multiculturalism signifies a preoccupation with race and gender—a preoccupation that allows just a whiff of class consciousness to sharpen the pungent odor of subjugation and resistance."[4]

Thus, for all the talk in some circles about the revival of regionalism and the immense popularity of such works as the *Encyclopedia of Southern Culture* (1989), regionalism remains low on the agenda of most American historians. One need only look at the quarterly bibliographies of "Recent Scholarship" that appear in the *Journal of American History* for proof. All four regional headings together—East, South, West, and Midwest—typically generate far fewer entries than, say, women's history or ethnic history, and more than 90 percent of the regional items focus on the West and the South. Recent surveys of the teaching of American history show that most regionally oriented courses also concentrate on the West and the South, although a few schools have lately instituted courses on the Rocky Mountain states.[5]

In this essay I explore the significance of regions in the history and historiography of American medicine. Rather than attempting a comprehensive survey of medical regionalism in the United States, or even of developments in a single region, I will present a wide-ranging series of examples that illustrate how medical historians have employed the concept of regionalism in their studies and show some of the many ways regional considerations have influenced the course of medicine in America. In this way I hope to suggest the fruitfulness, even the importance, of thinking regionally when writing about American medical history.

I have no interest in arbitrarily defining the meaning of *region*. For purposes of historical analysis, regions can be nodal or they can be uniform; they can be determined physiographically or culturally or epidemiologically—but never rigidly. For heuristic purposes, we may choose, for example, to focus our attention on the states lying between the Sierra Nevada and the Rocky Mountains, but as we shall see, few episodes in the medical history of the mountain West have been bounded by those precise geological structures, and some phenomena have even spilled across the international borders separating the United States from Canada and Mexico.

Although there is much to be learned from examining the medical culture of regions, we should guard against any trace of chauvinism or provincialism. Our goal as historians is not to celebrate the achievements of a region or to revel in antiquarian detail but to gain a better understanding of the role of place in history. We should also refrain from claiming uniqueness for a region until we first learn what transpired elsewhere. All too often, distinctiveness turns out to be an artifact of ignorance. With those caveats in mind, let us take a look at medical regionalism in America.

Despite a geographical tradition dating back to Hippocrates' treatise *On Airs,*

Waters, and Places and the dominance of regional thinking in nineteenth-century medicine, American medical historians have paid scant attention to regions. A few early works, such as Madge E. Pickard and R. Carlyle Buley's *The Midwest Pioneer: His Ills, Cures & Doctors* (1946) looked at medicine regionally—and discovered not only a common medical history in the Midwest but also "a distinct spirit of regional self-consciousness." However, most medical historians, when not looking at the national scene, have restricted their attention to particular cities or states. Because cities often led the fight against filth and disease, they have proved especially attractive to historians of public health. Even more medical historians have taken the state as their unit of analysis. Often this is done for chauvinistic reasons—to celebrate the anniversary of a state medical society, for example—but state analyses are not without value. After all, state legislatures have long determined the qualifications of health-care professionals, established boards of health to promote hygienic standards and combat disease, and regulated such activities as medical insurance, nursing homes, and the sale of drugs.[6]

No recent historian shows greater sensitivity to the importance of regional differences in medical theory and practice than John Harley Warner, a native southerner sensitive to the all-too-common habit of "overgeneralizing the experience of a single region, the Northeast." Warner's prize-winning book, *The Therapeutic Perspective* (1986), illustrates in rich detail the changing meaning of therapeutic regionalism in nineteenth-century America. "Early in the century," he writes, "the notion that the physical and social environments were significant factors in determining appropriate therapeutic behavior made region a necessary consideration in planning a patient's treatment and in evaluating the applicability of knowledge from another place, but by the 1880s therapeutic regionalism and nationalism had by and large become stigmata of inferior practice and antiquated thinking." Warner describes this change as a shift from specificity to universalism: from therapeutic judgments based on the peculiarities of a patient's race, class, gender, and place of residence to a reliance on knowledge increasingly generated in laboratories (perhaps even from experiments on animals) and applied indiscriminately to all humans, regardless of who they were or where they lived.[7]

Because of their allegiance to the doctrine of specificity, argues Warner, antebellum American physicians typically insisted on acquiring therapeutic knowledge in their own locales. "As surely as there is a distinction between foreign and American medicine," declared a New Orleans practitioner in the mid-1850s, "so surely is there a distinction between Northern and Southern medicine." One of the consequences of this belief was an often strident defense of regional medical education. Basic scientific knowledge might have universal applicability, but what sense did it make for, say, a southern medical student to learn about clinical practice in Paris, London, or Philadelphia when he intended to treat southern patients, with their peculiar diseases and constitutions? Although such notions transcended regional boundaries, southern medical educators, caught up in the intense sectional rivalries of the pre–Civil War period, took them to their farthest extreme.[8]

The doctrine of specificity also fostered research in medical geography. As Warner points out, "the notion that climate combined with other modifying influences to demand distinctively northern, southern, and western therapeutics was a cardinal corollary to the principle of specificity."[9] Some scholars Whiggishly characterize American medicine before the advent of the germ theory of disease as prescientific, but a century before Louis Pasteur and Robert Koch, numerous American physicians avidly investigated the links between climate and disease, hoping thereby to solve the mystery of etiology.

The epitome of this tradition is Daniel Drake's *Systematic Treatise, Historical, Etiological, and Practical, on the Principal Diseases of the Interior Valley of*

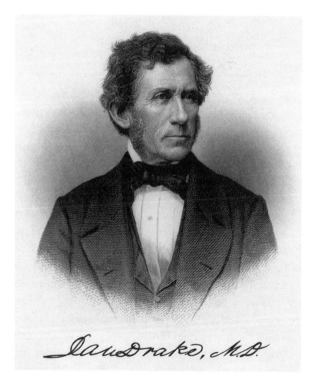

Daniel Drake, M.D. From *Pioneer Life in Kentucky: A Series of Reminiscential Letters from Daniel Drake, M.D., of Cincinnati, to His Children* (Cincinnati: Robert Clark, 1870), frontispiece.

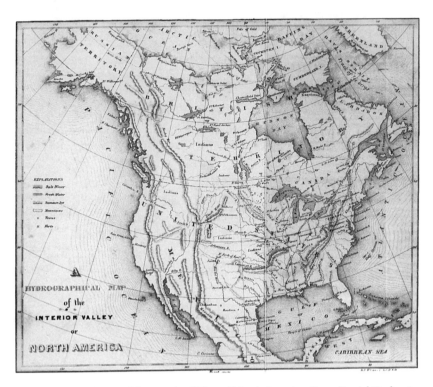

A hydrographical map of the Interior Valley of North America. From Daniel Drake, *A Systematic Treatise, Historical, Etiological, and Practical, on the Principal Diseases of the Interior Valley of North America* (Cincinnati: Winthrop B. Smith, 1850), frontispiece.

North America (1850, 1854). This monumental two-volume work surveys the distinctive disease patterns found in the "great intermontane region" between the Rockies and the Alleghenies, bounded on the north by the Polar Sea and on the south by the Gulf of Mexico. By identifying the geological, meteorological, and social determinants of disease—including diet, drink, and dress—the Cincinnati physician hoped to lay "the foundation of local medical history and practice" in this natural region. Drake explicitly defended a regional approach rather than a state or national one on the grounds that "civil divisions" were an inadequate basis for a study of the history of disease. "Physical causes lie at the bottom of whatever differences the maladies of different portions of the earth may present," he wrote; "and hence the region which a medical historian selects, should have well-defined natural, and not merely conventional boundaries." By assiduously collecting epidemiological data from throughout the region, Drake was able to establish the geographical limits of malaria (also known as intermittent fever), typhus (or continued fever), and yellow fever.[10]

If diseases are "the true actors in the history of medicine," as Erwin H. Acker-knecht liked to say, then regionally based histories make a great deal of sense.[11] Diseases, Daniel Drake noted, know no city limits or state lines—or even national borders. No region has attracted more attention from medical historians than the American South, whose very identity has sometimes centered on disease. The South long suffered from a well-deserved reputation for being the unhealthiest region in the nation, an area where strength and energy were sapped by the "Southern trilogy of 'lazy diseases'": malaria, hookworm, and pellagra. And long after yellow fever disappeared from the North, it continued to ravage the South and ultimately provided the impetus for public-health reform in the region. "Up until well into the twentieth century," writes the historian John Ett-ling, this "curious group of regional ailments held sway in the land below the Potomac, marking it off . . . as a country within a country."[12]

With the exception of pellagra, the South's most distinctive diseases—falci-parum malaria, hookworm, and yellow fever—all came from Africa in partial payment for the region's massive importation of slaves and struck African Americans with far less severity than whites. As K. David Patterson has recently shown, the prevalence of these diseases varied markedly throughout the South, creating not one but four distinctive disease environments, or epidemiological subregions: the Appalachian Mountains, which virtually escaped the diseases imported from Africa; the Atlantic Coastal Plain, which suffered greatly from malaria and hookworm but only sporadically from yellow fever; the Gulf Coast

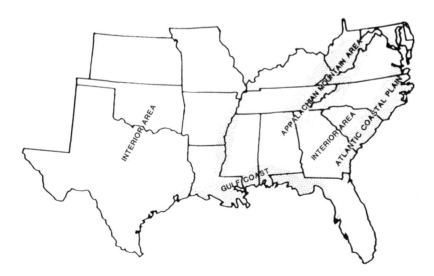

Epidemiological subregions of the southern United States before the Civil War. Courtesy of K. David Patterson.

and lower Mississippi Valley area, which was vulnerable to all three African diseases; and the remaining interior South, characterized by the absence of yellow fever and a relatively low incidence of malaria and hookworm.[13]

Not surprisingly, some of the best disease-oriented studies of American medicine have focused on the South: Elizabeth W. Etheridge on pellagra, John Ettling on hookworm, and Margaret Humphreys and John H. Ellis on yellow fever are examples.[14] But other sections have not been totally neglected. Half a century ago Ackerknecht wrote a pioneering regional history entitled *Malaria in the Upper Mississippi Valley* (1945), and recently Victoria A. Harden published an excellent history of Rocky Mountain spotted fever. Although the latter disease, a rickettsial infection carried by ticks, occurred throughout North America, the mountain West seemed especially vulnerable to it. Appropriately, laboratories in the Bitterroot Valley of Montana led the way in fighting the disease.[15]

Several authors have commented on the role of tuberculosis in the early history of the Rocky Mountain region. Almost from the beginning of European exploration, the salubrity of the mountains elicited favorable comment. George Frederick Ruxton, a young Englishman who explored in the vicinity of Pike's Peak in the spring of 1847, noted the "extraordinary fact that the air of the mountains has a wonderfully restorative effect upon constitutions enfeebled by pulmonary disease."[16] In the early 1860s, sometime silver prospector and western journalist Mark Twain discovered the curative powers of the region around Lake Tahoe. "Three months of camp life on Lake Tahoe would restore an Egyptian mummy to his pristine vigor, and give him an appetite like an alligator," he reported in his autobiographical account *Roughing It* (1872):

> I know a man who went there to die. But he made a failure of it. He was a skeleton when he came, and could barely stand. He had no appetite, and did nothing but read tracts and reflect on the future. Three months later he was sleeping out of doors regularly, eating all he could hold, three times a day, and chasing game over mountains three thousand feet high for recreation. And he was a skeleton no longer, but weighed part of a ton. This is no fancy sketch, but the truth. His disease was consumption. I confidently commend his experience to other skeletons.[17]

When word of the mountains' healing powers reached the East, hordes of consumptives—many of them physicians—began pouring into the Rocky Mountain region in search of a cure. And those who regained their health in the West shared their stories of salvation from sickness with evangelistic fervor. By 1880 an estimated one-third of the population of Colorado, nicknamed "The World's Sanitarium," consisted of health seekers and their families. The so-called lungers also played a central role in the social and medical history of New

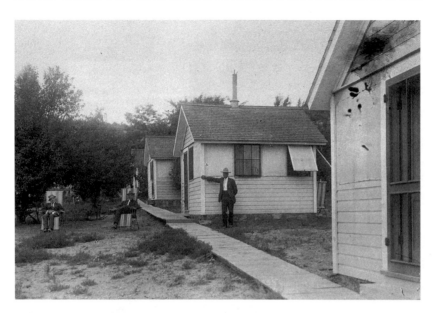

Cabins with canvas-flap windows for tuberculosis patients in New Mexico. Courtesy of New Mexico Medical History Archives. Also published in Jake W. Spidel Jr., *Doctors of Medicine in New Mexico: A History of Health and Medical Practice, 1886–1986* (Albuquerque: University of New Mexico Press, 1986), 121.

Mexico. Hundreds of tubercular physicians migrated to the state, and, as in Colorado, hospitals sprang up to meet the needs of the sick. For a while it was said that Albuquerque "had only two industries, the Santa Fe railroad and tuberculosis." Nevada and Utah similarly felt the effects of the white plague, although to a much lesser extent.[18]

For decades, altitude therapy, or climatotherapy, remained the treatment of choice for tuberculosis, at that time the nation's number one killer. At one point researchers claimed to have discovered a line of immunity, at about five thousand feet above sea level, above which tuberculosis germs could not survive. By the early twentieth century, however, physicians were turning increasingly to sanatoria as the first line of defense against the white plague. As the benefits of isolation and hospital care—wherever it was provided—became clear, more and more patients sought help in sanatoria close to home rather than trekking west for an expensive mountain cure. "By the time of World War II," writes Frank B. Rogers, "climatotherapy in the United States was a dead issue," ridiculed by the medical community as "a pseudo-science."[19]

Long before these developments, however, many residents of the mountain states had soured on the prospect of serving as the nation's sanatorium. For years regional boosters had been complaining that deadly tuberculosis germs

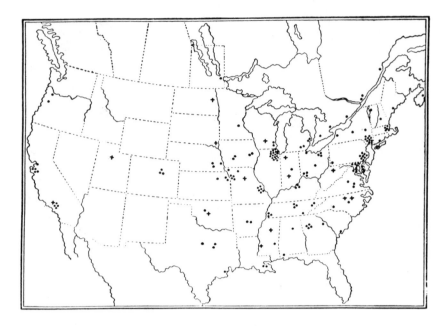

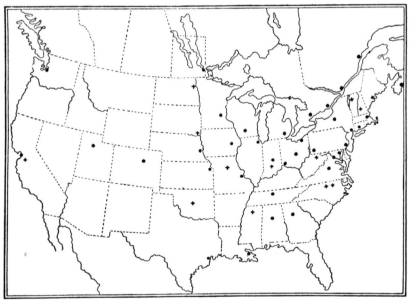

Maps showing (top) the actual number, location, and distribution of medical schools in the United States and Canada in 1910 and (bottom) the number, location, and distribution of medical schools recommended by Abraham Flexner in 1910. From Abraham Flexner, *Medical Education in the United States and Canada: A Report to the Carnegie Foundation for the Advancement of Teaching* (New York: Carnegie Foundation, 1910).

were polluting their pristine mountain environment, and employers had been openly discriminating against tuberculars. About the time of World War I, the affected states, from Kansas to California, banded together to appeal to the federal government to relieve them of the cost of caring for the many indigent sufferers who had relocated in the West. The former boon had now become a burden.[20]

Regional considerations have also had a profound effect on American medical education. As we have already seen, medical educators before the Civil War commonly employed the principle of specificity to justify therapeutic training in the region of intended practice. But regional considerations also played a role in the great reformation of medical education that occurred during the half century between the 1870s and the 1920s. In drawing his blueprint for the new system of medical education, Abraham Flexner, one of the chief architects of medical-school reform, used a regional template, arguing that sectional boundaries were of far greater importance than state lines. In his 1910 exposé of the pitiful condition of American medical schools, Flexner recommended reducing the number of institutions from 148 to 31, a move that would have eliminated 117 existing schools.[21]

In stark contrast to the rest of the nation, the entire mountain region boasted only two and a half medical schools: the Denver and Gross College of Medicine in Denver, the University of Colorado School of Medicine in Boulder, and the half school at the University of Utah in Salt Lake City. Denver and Gross was an amalgamated proprietary school nominally affiliated with the University of Denver. "Its equipment," reported Flexner, "consists of a chemical laboratory of the ordinary medical school type, a dissecting-room, containing a few subjects as dry as leather, a physiological laboratory with slight equipment, and the usual pathology and bacteriology laboratories." Although the college owned an "exceedingly attractive dispensary building," Flexner saw no reason to save it in view of the fact that Colorado was already overrun with physicians and did not need to produce many more. The University of Colorado was in much better shape, needing only to gain greater access to clinical material in Denver. Utah offered only two years of training in the basic sciences, but what Flexner saw, he liked.[22]

Given the region's relatively slow growth, Flexner calculated that it could safely absorb only about 120 new M.D.s a year, a quantity that two schools could easily produce. Besides, the region was still attracting physicians from other parts of the country, and some ambitious families preferred "sending their sons to Minneapolis, Madison, Ann Arbor, Chicago, or St. Louis." By the time Flexner's report appeared, the two Colorado schools had announced a merger, thus making the mountain region the first to come into compliance with Flexner's recommendations.[23]

After moving to the Rockefeller-funded General Education Board in 1912, Flexner drew on intraregional rivalries to stretch the Rockefeller dollars targeted for upgrading the training of American physicians. In the Midwest, for example, instead of underwriting the reorganization of several state medical schools, Flexner recommended giving funds only to the University of Iowa. "Knowing the spirit of emulation that prevailed throughout the West," he explained, "I felt sure that if the board helped to build and equip a thoroughly modern medical school in Iowa, other states would be constrained to follow suit out of their own resources . . . since no western state could afford to have it said that the University of Iowa possessed the best medical school in the Middle West." Sure enough, as soon as Iowa improved its faculty and facilities, neighboring state legislatures entered into a "friendly rivalry" to make sure that their own medical schools did not lag behind Iowa's.[24]

In the less competitive Northwest and mountain regions, medical educators proposed a number of cooperative plans for training physicians. In the early 1960s, for example, the Western Interstate Commission for Higher Education explored various ways to meet the medical-education needs of Idaho, Montana, Nevada, and Wyoming, none of which possessed so much as an internship or residency program, to say nothing of a medical school. For a time there was talk

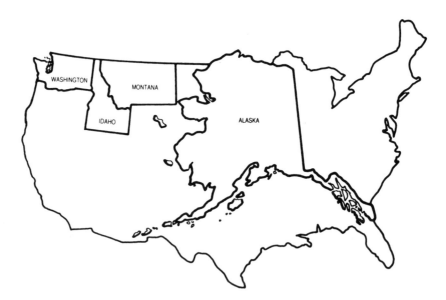

Logo of the University of Washington School of Medicine Primary Care Teaching Program, named WAMI for the states it served. From Nancy Rockafellar and James W. Haviland, eds., *From Saddlebags to Scanners: The First 100 Years of Medicine in Washington State* (Seattle: Washington State Medical Association, 1989).

of having the University of Utah medical school serve as a regional center for the five mountain states, but Utah lacked the ability to expand sufficiently to accommodate the needs of its neighbors. Besides, the states seemed to lack the regional solidarity necessary to make a cooperative plan work. "Despite many similarities, the four states of Idaho, Montana, Nevada, and Wyoming cannot accurately be described as a region, in either a geographic or an economic sense," noted one observer. "Each state is different and conscious of its differences." In the early 1970s Idaho and Montana joined with Alaska and Washington to form WAMI, a four-state network of teaching centers affiliated with the University of Washington medical school. Students from the four cooperating states could take their basic science courses in their home universities and then move to one of the WAMI facilities for clinical training, including, after the mid-1970s, residencies.[25]

Several years ago Daniel M. Fox introduced the phrase "hierarchical regionalism" to describe the dominant health-care policy in Britain and America during the period from 1911 to 1965. According to the advocates of this organizational scheme, medical knowledge would flow down from the laboratories of medical schools and teaching hospitals through lower-level institutions and on to the workaday physicians practicing in the surrounding regions. These health-care planners, including the majority on the Committee on the Costs of Medical Care in the early 1930s, believed that "geographic areas . . . rather than individual practices, clinics, or hospitals, are the proper units for which to plan, administer, and evaluate medical care." Unfortunately, Fox discussed only the rhetoric of regionalism; we still know little about hierarchical regionalism in action. Case studies of how this concept was implemented in particular regions, such as the mountain West, would be especially valuable.[26]

We do know that the U.S. Public Health Service carved the country into public-health districts in the early 1920s, and in 1965, in response to federal legislation calling for greater efforts to link medical research in the laboratory with medical care at the bedside, established the first Regional Medical Program (RMP). Within a few years more than fifty RMPs had been created.[27]

Although in many respects regional distinctions seem to be disappearing, striking differences—even within geographically similar regions—occasionally emerge. Nearly two decades ago the economist Victor R. Fuchs called attention to the remarkable health advantages the residents of Utah enjoyed over their neighbors in Nevada, despite both groups having similar incomes and access to health care. "The inhabitants of Utah are among the healthiest individuals in the United States," he noted, "while the residents of Nevada are at the opposite end of the spectrum." This was true even when the sin cities of Reno and Las Vegas were eliminated from the comparison. The key to explaining the differences, Fuchs concluded, was "the different life-styles of the residents of

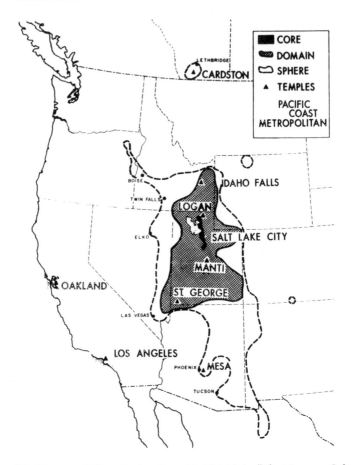

The Mormon Culture Region. From D. W. Meinig, "The Mormon Culture Region: Strategies and Patterns in the Geography of the American West, 1847–1964," *Annals of the Association of American Geographers* 55 (1965): 214.

the two states": "Utah is inhabited primarily by Mormons, whose influence is strong throughout the state. Devout Mormons do not use tobacco or alcohol and in general lead stable, quiet lives. Nevada, on the other hand, is a state with high rates of cigarette and alcohol consumption and very high indexes of marital and geographical instability. The contrast with Utah in these respects is extraordinary." Fuchs, relying on state statistics, understandably emphasized the differences between Utah and Nevada. But his argument would have been even more convincing, at least from a methodological point of view, had he contrasted the entire Mormon culture region with the surrounding areas. As the geographer D. W. Meining has argued, this region possesses "a *core* in the Wasatch Oasis, a *domain* over much of Utah and southeastern Idaho, and a *sphere* extending from eastern Oregon to Mexico" and even up to Alberta—a further reminder that regions often recognize no national boundaries.[28]

Few medical activities, especially in the Northwest and mountain areas, reflect regionalism more overtly than the organization of societies and the publication of journals. Medical societies typically embrace the physicians of a particular state, although some cross state lines. When the founders of the Colorado territorial medical society in 1871 overlooked their brethren in southern Colorado, those slighted physicians united with colleagues in northern New Mexico to form the short-lived, pretentiously named Rocky Mountain Medical Association. And in the 1930s, physicians in Colorado, Wyoming, New Mexico, and Utah, fearing encroachment by the federal government as well as by "cults and quacks," joined forces in the Rocky Mountain Medical Conference. "The past four years of depression have been a blessing to us," declared a Utah doctor in 1938, "because we were forced to fight for our own rights and for the health of our people. We learned to bury our petty differences and we now face the common foe unitedly. We are beginning to oppose crooked politicians and cultists who are securing wealth and power at the expense of public health."[29]

Reflecting this new sense of regional identity, the journal *Colorado Medicine*, which had long included the physicians of Wyoming as well as Colorado among its readers, renamed itself the *Rocky Mountain Medical Journal*. For years the journal served as the official publication of the medical societies of Colorado, Montana, Nevada, New Mexico, Utah, and Wyoming and promoted the study of "various diseases common to our Rocky Mountain region." In the mid-1970s Utah and Nevada bolted to sign on with the *Western Journal of Medicine,* a publication of the California Medical Association that aspired to become "a truly regional medical journal." By 1990 it was representing the state societies of Idaho, Nevada, New Mexico, Utah, and Wyoming, as well as the Denver Medical Society and several state societies in the far West.[30]

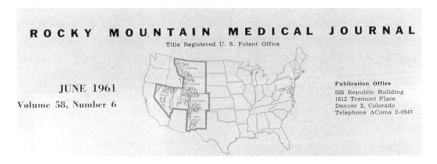

Logo of the *Rocky Mountain Medical Journal,* published in Denver, Colorado, 1961.

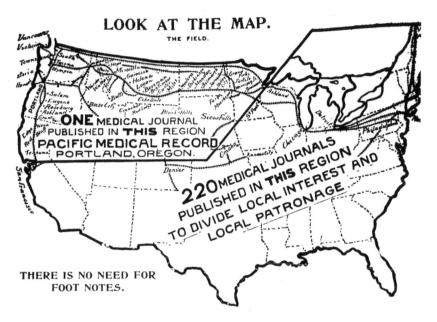

Advertisement for the *Pacific Medical Record. Pacific Medical Record* 1 (June–July 1893), inside front cover.

Regional medical journals in the mountain West date back to 1880 and the launching of the *Rocky Mountain Medical Review.* Although it lasted only two years under its original name, the *Review's* spirit survived various mergers and takeovers until 1933, when the *Western Medical Times,* its final incarnation, expired. Meanwhile the monthly *Pacific Medical Record,* an Oregon-based publication that quickly changed its name to the *Medical Sentinel,* was trying to establish itself as the medical journal of choice for the entire Northwest and upper mountain region. As the editor emphasized in justifying the appearance of his journal in 1893, the mammoth region west of Minneapolis–St. Paul and north of San Francisco and Denver supported only a single journal, in contrast to the 220 published elsewhere in the United States. Thus geographical remoteness, not "local pride," prompted his undertaking. "After all," he wrote, "the boundaries which nature has made, the geographical necessities of a region, determine to a great degree the needs of medical societies, colleges and journals." By the early twentieth century the *Sentinel* had established affiliations with the state medical societies of Oregon, Washington, Idaho, Montana, Wyoming, and Utah.[31]

I could go on and on reciting instances of the significance of regions in American medical history—from the popularity of contract practice in the antebellum South to the appeal of group practice in the Midwest, from missionary medicine in Catholic America to botanic medicine in Mormon America—but I think I have made my point.[32] Regions—whether geographical, cultural, or epidemiological—have been and continue to be a significant locus for medical activity in America. I am not arguing that historians should abandon writing about persons, communities, and states in favor of regions, or that we should privilege region over religion, race, class, or gender in our historical studies. And I am certainly not urging historians to celebrate the achievements of particular regions, no matter how much historical neglect these may have suffered. I am simply saying that medical historians should not overlook the significance of regional thinking and regional developments in writing about the American past, and I am suggesting that some medical-historical questions can be answered satisfactorily only in a regional context. As we should know by now, regionalism is not necessarily provincialism.

2 Steaming Saints

Mormons and the Thomsonian Movement

in Nineteenth-Century America

THOMAS J. WOLFE

Among the earliest nineteenth-century immigrants to settle in the intermountain West were members of the Church of Jesus Christ of Latter-day Saints (or LDS), commonly called the Mormons. Their exodus from the Midwest to escape persecution and their struggles to create agricultural oases in the harsh high deserts are familiar chapters in American history. Less well known, however, is that along with their distinctive religion the Mormons also carried westward an equally distinctive herbal medical system called Thomsonianism. The relation between Mormonism and Thomsonian medical practice stands as an interesting example of the interplay between medicine and religion in the West. Both groups, Mormons and Thomsonians, arose during the early republican period from similar political, religious, and social backgrounds. As we shall see, Thomsonian medical techniques, rhetoric, and ideology were well suited for adoption by the Mormons. At the same time, the religious sympathies of the Mormons for compatible Thomsonian views of medicine contributed to the continuation of Thomsonian practice in the American West long after the Thomsonian system had been abandoned in the rest of the country.

Samuel Thomson, the founder of the movement that would bear his name, was born in Alstead, New Hampshire, to a poor farm family in 1769. His parents were Massachusetts natives prompted by population pressure to move to the sparsely settled semifrontier of western New Hampshire. While still a young boy, Thomson became interested in the medicinal properties of plants and often accompanied a local healer, Mehitabel Benton, when she collected herbs; from her he learned about specific plants and their medical uses. For the most part, however, Thomson was self-taught as a medical practitioner.[1]

As a young adult Samuel set his hand to tending the family farm. Soon he married and began a family. Before long, however, he found himself thinking once again about herbal medicine—driven in part by his disgust with the mal-administrations of several physicians who had treated his wife and mother. Building on his earlier interests, Thomson began testing the effects of various plants and preparations. His crowning achievement, in his estimation, was the discovery of the emetic properties of *Lobelia inflata,* or Indian tobacco, which he considered crucial for the cure of disease.

Through trial-and-error therapeutics, Thomson gradually evolved a theoretical framework for understanding illness and its cure. Disease, he concluded, was caused by the loss of body heat. The human body was analogous to a steam engine; the stomach was the boiler. Medicines should "increase the internal heat, remove all obstruction to the system, restore the digestive powers of the stomach, and produce a natural perspiration."[2] Puking and peppering—lobelia to open up the system and cayenne pepper to rekindle the body's heat—formed the basis of Thomson's therapy. He completed his medical arsenal with additional herbs and distinctive vapor baths, which earned Thomsonians the sobriquet "steam doctors." His techniques stood in stark contrast to the practices of regular physicians, whose standard remedies included bloodletting and dosing with mineral-based drugs. In Thomson's view, these therapies did the patient more harm than good because they depleted the body of its natural heat.

Thomson's reputation as a healer spread from his family and friends to neighboring areas, and eventually even strangers approached him for advice or asked him to attend their families. By about 1805, he had given up farming and become a full-time healer, with much of New England as his territory. At the instigation of a jealous physician, a criminal charge of manslaughter was brought against him in 1809. Although he was acquitted, Thomson sought and received a U.S. patent on his botanic medical system in 1813, reasoning that federal approval would protect him from further malicious prosecutions.

Patent in hand, Thomson began to market his medical techniques on a broad scale. For $20, a purchaser received a so-called family right, which allowed personal and family use of Thomson's system; provided instruction in the form of Thomson's manual, *A New Guide to Health;* and enrolled the buyer in the Friendly Botanic Society. Before long, Thomsonians occupied a broad range of botanic medical practice from family right holders to full-time professionals. As interest grew, Thomson installed agents throughout the country to facilitate sales. A list from 1833 reveals the existence of 167 sales agents in twenty-one states and territories.[3] The *Medical Advocate,* published in Boston in 1827, was the first of more than sixty Thomsonian journals. In 1832, local Friendly Botanic Societies sent delegates to Columbus, Ohio, for the first United States Botanic Convention. The Thomsonians thus had a national organization some fifteen years before the American Medical Association was founded.[4]

From its New England roots, the Thomsonian movement had spread across the nation. In 1835, when Thomsonians claimed that half the residents of Ohio used the system, regular physicians responded that it was only one-third. That same year, the governor of Mississippi estimated that half of his state's citizens were Thomsonians. Thomsonians led organized legislative efforts to repeal medical licensing laws; by 1845 they could point to success in all but a few states. Their success cleared the way for an influx of other alternative medical systems. Hydropathy, homeopathy, eclectic medicine, and later osteopathy and chiropractic would all benefit from the formidable challenge to regular medicine posed by Samuel Thomson and his followers.

Marketing and organization alone do not explain the phenomenal success of the Thomsonian movement. Most attractive were Thomson's therapeutics, which exhibited an appealing naturalism in the idea that American plants were the only medicine required to treat American diseases. Obviously, then, nationalism also played a role in promoting the system. The prevailing political ideology of the period, republicanism, stressed ideals of self-reliance, virtue, and equality, and embraced as well a strong antimonopoly sentiment. Thomsonianism, with its message of self-help and suspicion of physicians who sought medical licensing, was well situated to benefit from such a climate. A Thomsonian slogan, "Every man his own physician," captures that spirit. Another reason for Thomson's success was the movement's conscious appeal for women's support at a time when the regular medical profession barred women from medical schools and was attempting to monopolize obstetrical practice. Thomson campaigned vociferously for the continued employment of midwives at births rather than physicians.[5]

To this diverse and complex mixture of factors promoting the popularity of the Thomsonian system can be added the subtle and intricate contribution of religion. More than thirty years ago, historian Charles Rosenberg, in his groundbreaking book *The Cholera Years,* suggested that medical and religious reformers often had a common cause.[6] My own findings reinforce this view and link many supporters of Thomsonianism to religionists who were challenging the established churches of the fledgling United States. In a database of nearly six thousand Thomsonians active around 1835, at least ninety-seven members of the clergy can be identified. Methodists were the largest group, followed by Baptists and a scattering of other religious affiliations.[7]

At the time the United States was founded, four denominations—Congregationalists, Anglicans (soon to be called Episcopalians), Presbyterians, and

Baptists—dominated the religious landscape and accounted for some 75 percent of all churches. The first three churches can be considered the "mainstream" of the period; many were so-called standing churches supported by tax money. The Baptists were the first in a wave of religious reformers bent on contesting the older churches that would later include the Methodists, Universalists, and sundry others. If the Baptists are excluded, the three remaining mainstream denominations still accounted for nearly 60 percent of all churches in 1780.[8] Among the ministerial Thomsonians, however, only four were Congregationalists, Episcopalians, or Presbyterians; the vast majority were affiliated with religious denominations that challenged the status quo. Clearly, a strong correlation existed between religious reform and medical reform. There are no Mormons on the list of ministerial Thomsonians because the Latter-day Saints did not sanction an official clergy separate from the church's male lay leadership.

Joseph Smith Jr., the founder of the LDS church, was born in Sharon, Vermont, less than fifty miles from Samuel Thomson's birthplace, on December 23, 1805. The Smith family's history mirrored that of the Thomsons. The same population pressures pushed Smith's grandfather, who was in the same generation as Thomson's father, to relocate his family from Massachusetts to western New England. Joseph Smith Sr. continued the westward movement, settling near Palmyra in upstate New York. Young Joseph probably received a little more education than most of the boys growing up in that time and place because both of his parents had been schoolteachers.[9]

Joseph's life changed dramatically at the age of fifteen when he received the first in a series of divine and angelic visitations. In his early twenties, Smith was allowed to take possession of a set of inscribed golden plates, which told the story of a group of Hebrews who escaped Jerusalem before the Babylonian invasion and eventually inhabited North America until their destruction in the fifth century A.D. The story became an essential part of the Book of Mormon, which was first published in 1830, the same year that Smith formally organized the Church of Jesus Christ of Latter-day Saints.

From its beginning the LDS church was extremely hierarchical, with tiers of elders, priests, teachers, and deacons. Within a few years fifteen men sat at the apex of the church: the three-man First Presidency, which consisted of the president, Joseph Smith, and two counselors; and the Quorum of Twelve Apostles. At the end of the church's first year of existence, its membership amounted to about 70 Mormons in New York and another 130 in Ohio. Proselytizing was a central mission for the new church, and it paid nearly immediate dividends when an entire congregation of Campbellite Disciples of Christ in Kirtland, Ohio, converted. In 1831, in the face of growing opposition and violence from their neighbors, Smith and most of the New York Saints moved to Kirtland. This was the beginning of a divinely revealed gathering of the Saints in a restored Zion. As church membership increased, the neighbors again grew uneasy, and then openly hostile, and church members moved to several successive locations in Missouri. In 1839, both Kirtland and Missouri were abandoned for Nauvoo, Illinois, on the Mississippi River.

In Nauvoo, the church continued to grow; by 1844, some eleven thousand members had congregated there. The same pattern of intensifying hostility and violence against the Mormons recurred. Smith was jailed and then murdered by a mob in June 1844, and leadership of the church passed to Brigham Young, the president of the Quorum of Twelve Apostles. It was Young who organized and led the Mormon exodus to present-day Utah.

Two features of historic Mormonism are probably best known today—the practice of polygamy and the hygienic proscriptions against caffeine, alcohol, and tobacco—yet neither was part of the original teachings of the church. Instead, Joseph Smith preached a divinely authorized mission to restore primitive Christianity, to bring back a pure church unencumbered by centuries of theological teachings. Smith's message of a restored gospel embodied in the Book of Mormon appealed to the many souls seeking comfort and certainty amid the religious cacophony that characterized the period. Indeed, historians have referred to upstate New York as the "burned-over district" because of the many revivals that swept through the area during the middle of the nineteenth century. Continuing revelations by Smith bolstered the foundation and uniqueness of the church.

Smith prophesied throughout his life, and his subsequent revelations, now known as the Doctrine and Covenants, form the second major document, after the Book of Mormon, supporting the LDS church. A discussion of Mormons and health care usually begins with this work. In 1833, Smith revealed the teaching now called the "Word of Wisdom" (Doctrine and Covenants, section 89), which is the basis for the present-day abstention from coffee, tea, alcohol, and tobacco. For most of the nineteenth century, however, abstention was a goal, not a commandment. In fact, Brigham Young officially advised Mormon pioneers to include coffee, tea, and alcohol among their supplies. Prescriptively, the "Word of Wisdom" advocated the consumption of herbs, fruits, vegetables, and wheat, and called for the sparing consumption of meat. Such prescriptions were not unique to the Mormons. Similar dietary advice was advocated by contemporary health reformers such as William Alcott, uncle of the novelist Louisa May, and Sylvester Graham, who is still renowned for his cracker.[10]

The Mormons recognized that healthful living would not eradicate disease. Illness could visit the faithful for a number of reasons: as chastisement, as an opportunity for the exhibition of God's healing power, as a test of faith, or as possession. As a result, faith healing has a long tradition among the Mormons. Many afflicted Mormons linked cures to the laying on of hands, rebaptism, anointing with oil, and, of course, blessings and prayers. Mormons could point to instances of faith healing in both the Bible and the Book of Mormon. If the LDS church was indeed the restored church, then successful faith healing was both a boon and a sign of confirmation.

At the time the LDS church was formed, Joseph Smith's attitude toward physicians bordered on contempt. Like Thomson, he and his family had experienced several questionable episodes while in the care of regular physicians. Of particular importance was the death in 1823 of his brother, Alvin, from calomel (a widely administered mercurial compound) that lodged in his intestines and caused gangrene.[11]

After leading his contingent of New York Saints to Kirtland, Smith initially stayed in the home of a recent convert, Frederick Granger Williams, a Thomsonian physician. Williams, a former teacher, farmer, and Lake Erie pilot, had bought a Thomsonian family right about 1821. Like some other Thomsonians, Williams began to practice professionally after he became adept at using the system, eventually assuming the title "doctor." By the time he became acquainted with Smith, Williams had built an extensive practice. To Williams goes the credit for introducing Smith to the distinctive therapeutics and ideology of Thomsonianism.[12] For Smith and other members of the early LDS church, Thomsonianism resonated with sympathetic themes. One of the most important was the Mormons' vision of their church as the restored primitive church, a view that connects Mormon attitudes toward Thomsonian practice with Methodist sympathies for the same therapies.

The sizable presence of Methodists within the Thomsonian movement was not by chance. John Wesley, the British founder of Methodism, had very specific views on medicine, which he expressed in *Primitive Physic*, one of the most popular medical guides of the eighteenth and early nineteenth centuries. "Primitive" in this context did not mean backward or ignorant; rather, Wesley was calling for a restoration of medicine to ordinary people, for a return to a simpler time when healing was a folk tradition based on experience and native human intelligence. Wesley attributed much of the disease and suffering evident in his time to the imposition of convoluted and perverted theories by "learned" physicians. Thomson and his followers were aware of Wesley's argument and adopted it nearly wholesale. Thomsonian medicine was cast as the return to the medicine of the ancients. Undoubtedly many Methodists, members of the fastest growing church in the early nineteenth-century United States, were drawn to Thomsonianism. The message was equally obvious to Joseph Smith and the Mormons, and it clearly complemented their own belief that they were participating in a religious restoration.[13]

It is not surprising, then, that many of the thirty-four men who held the top leadership positions in the LDS church—the First Presidency and Quorum of Twelve Apostles—from 1832 to 1849 were former Methodists. Historian D. Michael Quinn examined this group and was able to locate the prior denominations of thirty of the thirty-four. A full third were Methodists; if the eight men that Quinn identified as previously unchurched are eliminated, then the figure rises to 45 percent—far more than any other denomination.[14]

The mere fact that Methodists were well represented among both Thomsonians and the Mormon hierarchy does not prove, of course, that Thomsonians were well represented among the Mormons; but there is more direct evidence for a strong relationship. Less than a year after Smith met Frederick Williams, the man responsible for introducing him to Thomsonian medicine, Smith appointed Williams a counselor in the First Presidency and one of the high priests of the church. In addition, Williams served for more than three years as Smith's scribe and sermon writer. At the same time he continued to practice medicine, adding Smith and other prominent Mormons to his clientele.

Nor was Frederick Williams the sole Thomsonian in the highest circles of the church. The most prominent of all were the Richards brothers, Willard and Levi. The brothers converted to Mormonism in 1836 after reading the Book of Mormon (given to them by their cousin, Brigham Young) and then visiting with Smith in Kirtland. Although five years apart in age—Levi was born in 1799, Willard in 1804—the brothers apparently always followed similar interests. When Levi studied mechanics and science, so did Willard; both became school-teachers; both became interested in medicine after a sister died around 1830 from a mysterious illness that her physicians could not diagnose. Thereafter, both became Thomsonian practitioners and continued to practice, at least sporadically, as they moved up the church hierarchy. Levi replaced Frederick Williams as Joseph Smith's personal physician in 1837. At about the same time, he also advanced to become a high priest. A few years later, when the church was residing in Nauvoo, Smith saw to it that Levi was elected to the city council. When the legislature authorized a Mormon militia unit, the Nauvoo Legion, Levi became its surgeon general. He continued to hold important positions in the church throughout his life.[15]

Willard played an even more central role in the history of the church than Levi. He was a member of the first proselytizing mission to Great Britain, and while there he was appointed to the Quorum of Twelve Apostles. When he returned in 1841, he became Joseph Smith's private secretary; a short time later he became the church's historian and clerk. Willard was a prisoner along with Smith when the founder was murdered. As the only Apostle in the area at the time, Willard temporarily took control of the church until Brigham Young could assume the presidency. In 1847, Young named Willard a counselor in the

First Presidency, a position he held for the rest of his life. Once the Mormons had settled in Salt Lake City, Willard added the editorship of the official church newspaper, the *Deseret News,* to his ecclesiastical duties. Over the years, he occasionally used this pulpit to support Thomsonian medicine.[16]

Other Thomsonians joined the ranks of the Mormons and played roles both acclaimed and infamous in the history of the church. Avard Sampson, for example, formed a quasi-military band of raiders to exact revenge on suspected anti-Mormon persecutors during the Missouri sojourn of the church. He was excommunicated. At least six other professional Thomsonian practitioners treated fellow Mormons at Nauvoo or during the early Salt Lake years, including a woman named Margaret Cooper West. As the system was intended primarily for domestic use, undoubtedly many more church members utilized Thomson's remedies without being publicly recognized as Thomsonian healers.[17]

While Thomsonians were rife within the early church, only three regular physicians seem to have joined during those first years. Two were soon excommunicated, leaving Thomsonians in the best position to have an impact on the church and its medical philosophy.

In 1831, after arriving in Kirtland, Joseph Smith revealed that disease need not be treated by faith healing alone. "And whosoever among you are sick," he wrote, "and have not faith to be healed, but believe, shall be nourished with all tenderness with herbs and mild food."[18] Commentators interpreted this as an implicit endorsement of Thomsonian botanic medicine. Both the Bible and the Book of Mormon mention herbal remedies, and these provided additional warrants. In 1834, Smith more explicitly endorsed herbal medicine. At a church meeting he decreed: "And if there are any that believe that roots and herbs administered to the sick, and all wholesome vegetables which God has ordained for the use of man and if any say that such things applied to the sick in order that they may receive health, and this applied by any member of the Church, if there are any among you that teach that these things are of Satan, such teaching is not of God." Herbal medicine had the prophet's approval.[19]

It should be noted that there is no evidence that Smith ever endorsed Thomsonianism by name. Nevertheless, whether called botanic, herbal, or Thomsonian, the system was the quasi-official medicine of the church. During the Nauvoo period in the 1840s, Mormon botanic practitioners were "called" and "set apart" by church leaders to treat illness within the community. A municipal botanic board of health was also established during the Nauvoo years.[20]

Perhaps the most telling evidence for the importance of herbal medicine to the Mormons occurred after the exodus to Utah. In 1852, the territorial legislature launched an attack on regular medicine and passed a law that made it illegal for anyone—doctor, apothecary, or layperson—to dispense, counsel, or advise to another person any substance deemed to be poisonous without completely explaining to the "patient and surrounding friends and relatives" the "nature, operation and design" of the substance and then gaining the "full and free assent of said patient and friends." Offenders were guilty of a high misdemeanor, punishable by a fine of at least $1,000 and a minimum sentence of one year of hard labor. The law enumerated the proscribed substances: mercury, arsenic, antimony, or any preparations using the same; nightshade, opium, henbane, chloroform, ether, and laughing gas. A significant proportion of the regular physician's materia medica thus stood restricted, while the remedies of the botanics were unmentioned. Significantly, both Levi and Willard Richards were members of the legislature.[21]

In 1849, Thomsonians in Salt Lake City formed the Council of Health, whose initial purpose, according to William Morse, one of the founders, was to promote "the superiority of botanic practice." The council examined local plants for potential use as medicaments. Soon the council expanded its role and welcomed women members. With a reported membership of three hundred, the council directed much of its activity toward the training of midwives. So successful was the Council of Health that Priddy Meeks, a Thomsonian practitioner and council founder, reported: "Old Dr. Cannon, a 'poison' [regular] doctor, and poisoned against the Mormons too, could get but little to do among the sick; said if we would give him all the surgery to do he would quit doctoring; and so we did and he joined the Council of Health and proved a great benefit to us."[22] Dr. Cannon's difficulties were reflected in a survey of Salt Lake City medical practitioners who signed death certificates during the years 1847–71. Only six of thirty-five held the M.D. degree.[23]

Utah was the last bastion of Thomsonianism. Samuel Thomson died in 1843. His son and successor, John, survived him by only a few years. By then, the movement had already splintered into two camps. Professional practitioners with ambitions for Thomsonian medical schools and associations with licensing powers were arrayed against those who adhered to Thomson's original vision of self-help medicine. Under this stress and without effective leadership, Thomsonianism seemed to fade away by the end of the 1840s—except in Utah, where it enjoyed the sanction of the Church of Jesus Christ of Latter-day Saints.[24]

Herbal medicine persisted as a folk tradition among some Mormons in the mountain region for many years. As recently as the 1950s, folklorist Austin Fife found that "canker" was considered an indicator of a "basic bodily disturbance," and treatments featured infusions of bayberry bark. The same condition and treatment are described in Samuel Thomson's *New Guide to Health*.[25]

Besides the factors already mentioned, the persistence of Thomsonian and herbal medicine among the Mormons was also the result of another element, one especially deserving of attention because it highlights one of the main themes of this volume—namely, place. The Mormons settled in the remote mountain West so that the geography of the region could act as a bulwark against persecution. This self-enforced physical isolation served to bolster Thomsonian medical practice. Self-reliance was more than a virtue in Utah, it was a necessity. Instead of spending their scarce and hard-won cash on costly imported medicines, the Saints could simply plant and harvest many of their medical supplies.

Similarly, the isolation retarded the importation of new ideas and trends from the East. Nevertheless, new ideas and trends did eventually arrive; and so too did the transcontinental railroad after the Civil War. Increasingly, young Mormons traveled east to attend regular medical schools. By the turn of the century, Thomsonianism had all but disappeared from Utah.

So far, this paper has focused on the Mormons' involvement with Thomsonianism. How did non-Mormon Thomsonians react to that involvement? Only one piece of direct evidence has been found, and it expresses hostility toward the Mormons. The lack of comment in the Thomsonian press is undoubtedly due to the general public attitude toward the Latter-day Saints at that time. Many of their contemporaries viewed the early Mormons as extremely bizarre, even dangerous, especially after the secret practice of polygamy became public knowledge in the 1840s. Certainly many Thomsonians would have felt the same way. Thomsonian leaders were striving to have their system accepted by mainstream society at the time, and any connection between the Thomsonian movement and Mormonism was probably suppressed and denied.

The single discussion of Mormonism in a Thomsonian journal involves the curious case of Dr. John Cook Bennett, one of the two M.D.s excommunicated by the early LDS church. In retaliation, Bennett publicized the still secret practice of plural marriage in 1842. A few years later, when a Thomsonian medical school announced Bennett's appointment to its faculty, a letter appeared in a Thomsonian periodical excoriating Bennett for both his Mormon past and his regular physician background:

> Is there a father, or guardian—*unless he be of the "chosen of Nauvoo"*—who would like for his son or ward to listen daily to the immaculate Bennett, and thus have his mind impregnated with the hellish revelations of Mormonism, as well as *medical science?* . . . let every Thomsonian strive to heave from our ranks this *unseemly stone*. What! is there an affinity between Thomsonism and Mormonism? No. The union of these principles will form a compound that will prove destructive to Medical reform.[26]

The early Church of Jesus Christ of Latter-day Saints and the Thomsonian movement had many similarities. The founders of both groups came from westward-moving Massachusetts families. Both drew their original followers from members of that same group. Especially appealing to both groups was the similar message each preached of restoration. Indeed, some Mormons considered Thomson nearly as divinely inspired as Joseph Smith. As Thomsonian practitioner and Mormon Priddy Meeks put it:

> Then we should look on those principles [of Thomsonian practice] as an appendix to the gospel [the Book of Mormon] as a temporal salvation. It was introduced nearly contemporary with the gospel and in its main features runs in sympathy with the gospel, even the "Word of Wisdom" and Thomsonian[ism] run together and strengthen each other instead of coming in collision with each other.
>
> Thomson was educated the same as Joseph Smith was. . . . They tried to kill him the same as Joseph Smith; they lanced him the same as they did Joseph Smith and did everything in their power to stop its progress, but could not do it because it was of inspiration and, of course, of divine origin like Joseph Smith's mission.[27]

The Mormons were not a demographically significant group during the heyday of the Thomsonian movement. Nevertheless, their experience with Thomsonianism adds dimension to a larger question concerning how medicine and religion sometimes interact to challenge established orthodoxies.

3   Suicide in the Nevada Hinterlands

A Cultural Perspective

Suicide can be considered as a regional phenomenon in large areas of the mountain West. In 1991, for example, the suicide rate in the states of the mountain West far exceeded the nationwide figure of 12.2 per 100,000 population. Nevada led with a rate of 24.8 per 100,000 population, followed by Montana with 19.9, Wyoming with 18.9, New Mexico with 18.3, Arizona with 17.7, Colorado with 16.7, Utah with 16.2, and Idaho with 15.9.[1]

According to historian Sally Zanjani, the high rate of suicide in Nevada has deep roots in the history of the state.[2] Zanjani points out, for example, that John Wesley Powell noted a tradition of suicide among elderly Southern Paiute women in his early travels; and Marion Goldman noted a generally elevated suicide rate on the nineteenth-century Comstock and an "almost unbelievable" rate among the prostitutes she studied. Zanjani herself notes that "around the turn of the century when central reporting of mortality statistics began, Nevada suicides for 1910 were 3.9 percent of total mortality, while the national figure for 1906 was 0.9 percent."[3] Since the early 1900s, the gap has narrowed between Nevada and the rest of the nation, but in 1994 the state rate of 27.1 suicides per 100,000 population was still more than double the national rate, 12.4, and still the highest in the United States.[4]

The few investigators who have studied suicide in Nevada during the past twenty years have attempted to assess factors that might contribute to Nevada's high rates by focusing on the more notorious of the socioeconomic elements that set the state apart from the rest of the country. The explanation most commonly given (especially in the popular domain) is Nevada's sixty-year history of economic dependence on legalized gambling, which gives rise to twenty-four hour communities with easy access to alcohol, legalized prostitution, and "quickie" divorces, and a large tourist and transient population.[5] In a general book on suicide published under the auspices of the Unitarian Universalist Association in 1971, for example, Earl Grollman writes that Nevada "has an extremely high [suicide] rate due to gambling losses and a large transient population. The personally unhappy, the occupationally dissatisfied, the seekers after Nirvana go not only to Nevada but to California to seek contentment."[6] The perspective of one Nevada woman is typical: "Oh, all those people gamble away their money and then kill themselves."[7]

The extent to which gambling and the related tourist trade influence Nevada's suicide rate is difficult to assess. In an attempt to approach this problem, the Centers for Disease Control (CDC) conducted a brief study in 1989 and analyzed the suicide rate for visitors to Nevada during 1986–87.[8] The investigators found that the suicide rate for the two-year period was 15.8 per 100,000 visitor-years, a figure similar to the U.S. rate. This suggests that in spite of the daily loss of millions of gambling dollars, visitors to Nevada do not appear to be at higher risk than the rest of the U.S. population. The CDC investigators also found, however, that gaming industry employees, a large group of workers peculiar to the state of Nevada, had a rate of 43 per 100,000—a figure significantly higher than that for the state as a whole. Most gaming employees reside in the state's two largest urban areas, Reno-Sparks and Las Vegas. The socioeconomic makeup of the rest of Nevada presents a different picture that must also be considered, however. Furthermore, Nevada's suicides must be considered within the context of the entire mountain region.

Nevada's population of just over one million people is dispersed in a pattern as unique as the state's economy.[9] There is a sharp contrast between the vast, sparsely populated areas of rural Nevada and the urban centers of Las Vegas in Clark County and Reno-Sparks in Washoe County where 83 percent of the population lives. When the CDC investigators compared the suicide rates in Nevada's rural and urban areas, they found the age-adjusted rates to be similar except for urban females, who had a rate 50 percent higher than that of their rural counterparts.[10] It is important to note, however, that in 1989, 221 of the 303 suicides in Nevada occurred in the two urban counties (66 in Washoe County and 155 in Clark County) according to the *Nevada Vital Statistics Report*. Thus, 73 percent of the state's suicides occurred in areas where 82 percent of the population resided. This means that 27 percent of the suicides occurred where 18 percent of the population lived—in rural areas. These figures suggest that the rural areas may be contributing more than their fair share of suicides. In other words, suicides do not seem to be random with respect to residence: a totally random suicide distribution would correlate more closely with the population distribution.

The epidemiological studies discussed above have outlined the problem of suicide in Nevada but cannot fully reveal the cultural context and cultural patterns associated with suicide. I argue in this paper that a fuller cultural "scripting" of the act of suicide is needed to understand the phenomenon in the contexts of both Nevada and the larger mountain West. My assumption is that, aside from being a singular act, suicide expresses a larger cultural construction of its meaning. I focus on suicide in one rural community, White Pine County, Nevada, because the narrow frame of a single community provides a sharper image of the importance of the cultural construction of suicide. It is also easier to illuminate sociological and psychological phenomena and environmental dimensions that articulate with and inform the cultural context in a single-community study. Applying a cultural perspective to the study of suicide in rural Nevada may uncover historically rooted perceptions of life and death that color attitudes throughout the population.

I begin with a brief discussion of my methodology, which is followed by an ethnographic sketch of White Pine County. I then offer a profile of those individuals who seem most at risk for suicide in this community and compare this profile with the profile compiled by the CDC. This is followed by a discussion of themes or patterns of meaning having to do with the "intent" of the act of suicide by individuals. The paper ends with the argument that attitudes and feelings about the act of suicide are culturally constructed, and one must search within the elements of culture to understand suicide.[11]

I began my field research on community perceptions of health problems in White Pine County, Nevada, in the winter of 1991. I lived in Ely, the county seat of White Pine County, for three months (February–April 1991) and have since returned on three occasions for stays of several days. Although my original intent was to assess overall health problems, I quickly became alerted to the special issue of suicide. When queried in various university courses, students from White Pine County had reported to me their belief that suicide was one of the major health problems of the area, especially among young people. Preliminary research in the county also indicated that the community as a whole perceived suicide to be a notable problem. It thus seemed imperative to collect reliable data on suicide in the county.

I took data from death certificates issued from 1950 to 1990 that listed the cause of death as suicide (if doubt was indicated concerning suicide as the cause of death, the certificate was not included in the database). These data were supplemented with information from local newspaper articles (which were often very detailed) and obituaries written about the suicide victims. The local coroner's reports on the suicides, including actual suicide notes, were a third source of data. During this phase of my research I did not initiate interviews with family members of suicide victims, although on many occasions family members and others in the community initiated conversations with me and spoke openly of individual suicides.

The information I gathered indicates that there were 110 suicides during the forty-one-year period from 1950 to 1990. There are discrepancies between my figures and those listed in the *Nevada Vital Statistics Report* as to the number of annual suicides in White Pine County. My numbers are generally higher. I cannot account for the discrepancies except to say that I used data that I collected within the community. The investigators in the 1989 CDC study in Nevada noted the considerable controversy in the suicide literature regarding the validity of official vital statistics data and their use in the study of suicide.[12] As many as 50 percent of suicides may not be reported as such. Underreporting of suicides probably varies from area to area; no evidence of systematic overreporting has been published. Given this controversy, the CDC investigators examined the sensitivity to suicide as the mode of death, as indicated on the death certificates used in their study, and found it to be somewhere between 84 percent and 98 percent. They concluded that the mode of death is accurately reported on Nevada death certificates.

Some people have suggested to me that in relatively small communities, where most of the people know one another, suicides are not always reported because of the associated stigma, and that this might be especially true in communities with a substantial Mormon population, like White Pine County. I would argue that it would be very difficult to cover up or hide a suicide in White Pine County precisely because of the closeness of the community. The reported rate might be higher if officials could prove suspicions that particular vehicle accidents or other seemingly accidental events were in fact suicide.

White Pine County is close to nine thousand square miles in area and is sparsely settled. In 1989 the population density was 1.01 persons per square mile. (Because of this low population density, White Pine County is classified as a "frontier" county by public health officials, as compared with a "rural" county.) The majority of the county's population lives in Ely, the county seat and the largest community within a 240-mile radius. Within a few miles are the small communities of Ruth and McGill. This cluster of three communities sits at the end of what *Life* magazine in July 1986 designated "The Loneliest Road in America." Reno is 315 miles away, Las Vegas is 245 miles, and Salt Lake City, Utah, is 250 miles away.

The population of White Pine County has fluctuated drastically between

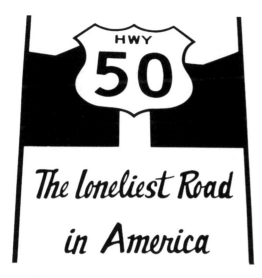

U.S. Highway 50, "The Loneliest Road in America."
From photo by Marie Boutté.

growth and decline. Over the past sixty years, the county experienced a population maximum of 12,377 in 1940 and a minimum of 7,640 in 1985. Between
1970 and 1980 the county lost nearly 2,000 people, the majority in the late 1970s
when the Kennecott Copper Company (the major industry in the area at that
time) shut its open-pit mine in Ruth. Others left when the company shut down
its smelting operation in McGill in 1983. In 1989 the population of White Pine
County climbed to almost 9,000 as a result of several recent economic boosts.[13]
In 1987, Nevada's first national park, the Great Basin National Park, was created
some sixty miles from Ely, the closest city of any size. This has increased
tourism in the area, as has the "Old Ghost Train of Old Ely," which takes visitors on short summer excursions from the railroad museum. A maximum security prison that can house close to a thousand inmates and provide employment for three hundred to four hundred permanent personnel was opened in
1990. There continues to be talk and hope that the White Pine Power Project,
which was projected to help solve the economic woes of the county, will be constructed, but the project appears to be in limbo. The search for low-grade gold
stimulates sporadic mining in the White Pine area.

White Pine County has historically been a mining community, beginning in
1865 with silver and then, after 1904, with copper. Since 1983 most of the mining in the area has been for gold. The towns of McGill, Ruth, and Ely were essentially company towns. In 1973, mining was by far the leading employer in
White Pine County, accounting for 28.3 percent of all wages and salaried posi-

tions; ten years later mining accounted for only 14.8 percent of wage and salary employment. In the early 1990s, tourist-related and retail businesses and government employment in the prison, the Forest Service, the Bureau of Land Management, and the local government and school district employed more individuals than mining, although mining still accounted for 19 percent of the workforce in 1991.

All of the mining efforts in White Pine County have undergone cycles of boom and bust. There is some evidence that such cycles influence the suicide rate. For example, there were six suicides in the county in 1984, when the unemployment rate was close to 18 percent, and seven in 1976, when unemployment was also high. There were eight suicides in White Pine County in 1992; in June 1992 the county led the state in unemployment with a jobless rate of 9.0 percent. (Statewide, the unemployment rate was 6.6 percent.) The *Reno Gazette-Journal* announced in mid-August 1992 that seventy-four people were being laid off from the Magma Nevada Mining Company because gold mining operations in the area were being curtailed.[14] Another seventy-four workers added to an already high number of unemployed in a small area constitutes a large increase. More research is needed to determine the relationship of unemployment to suicide rate, but a better understanding of the demographics and sociocultural context of White Pine County will also help to shed light on the county's suicide rate.

Some comparisons can be made between the demographic profiles of suicide victims in White Pine County and the state as a whole, although such comparisons are imperfect because they compare data from different time frames. According to the 1989 *Nevada Vital Statistics Report,* of 303 suicides in the state, 256 (84.5 percent) were males and 47 (15.5 percent) were females. There were 110 suicides in White Pine County during the forty-one-year period I examined; 92 percent were males and 8 percent were females. The White Pine data support the CDC findings that males are the highest-risk group and that urban females have a much higher suicide rate than their rural counterparts. Two interesting questions arise: Why the difference in rates between urban and rural females? And why are rural women not committing suicide in numbers even somewhat comparable to rural men?

There has long been concern about youth suicide in Nevada. In 1989, however, teenage suicides accounted for only 6.6 percent of all suicide deaths; adults 35 and older made up 59.4 percent.[15] From 1968 to 1989, the largest age group was 25–34, with 22.5 percent; followed by age group 45–54, with 17 percent. In White Pine County from 1950 to 1990, adults 35 and older committed 58.6 percent of suicides—about the same as the state rate for 1989, but the specific age categories are different. The largest age group in White Pine County was 55–64 years old, with 19 percent of the suicides; followed by age group 35–44, with

17.3 percent. Teenagers accounted for 10.9 percent, a number slightly higher than the statewide rate.

The CDC study suggests that divorced and widowed persons are at highest risk for suicide both in Nevada and in the United States as a whole. Married persons are at lowest risk, and never married people have an intermediate risk. In White Pine County between 1950 and 1990, 55 percent of suicides were married; 45 percent were either never married, divorced, widowed, or unknown.

The most common method of suicide in Nevada in 1989 was by firearms (63.7 percent), followed by drugs (11.6 percent) and hanging (11.2 percent).[16] The CDC investigators found that nearly 70 percent of the more than two thousand suicides in Nevada from 1978 to 1987 used firearms. In White Pine County, firearms accounted for 69 percent of the suicides during my forty-one-year research period; the second most common method was carbon monoxide (12.7 percent); hanging was third (8.2 percent). Thus, the vast majority of both urban and rural suicides favored firearms, but there was a rural-urban difference in the use of carbon monoxide versus drugs.

As discussed above, White Pine County has a fairly diverse economic base. I classified twenty-two discrete occupations among the 110 suicides, but several stand out in terms of suicide rates. Miners formed the largest percentage of suicides (25 percent), followed by students, construction workers, and government employees (7.3 percent in each category); and then ranchers, retirees, and self-employed (6.4 percent in each category). In contrast, gaming industry employees had the highest suicide rate in urban areas. Eighty percent of the 110 suicides in White Pine County were residents of the county; all but 8 were Caucasians of European heritage (3 were American Indians, 2 were of Asian heritage, and 3 were of Spanish heritage).

Who is at highest risk for suicide in White Pine County? The evidence shows that all males are at risk. But at greatest risk is a middle-aged or older Caucasian male who is a resident of the county, married, and once or presently employed in mining; he will most likely kill himself with a gun, and, according to suicide notes, he may be suffering from ill health.

This profile is similar in some but not all respects to the CDC profile for the highest-risk groups in the state. The CDC profile specifies males, both whites and nonblack minorities, widowed or divorced, and in certain employment categories (blue collar and gaming) as being at highest risk for suicide.

What is the meaning of suicide for the profiled individual I have described? How does he define or perceive the situation that leads him to take his own life? I believe that themes or patterns of meaning, in particular cognitive or "situated" meanings having to do with the "intent" of the act by the individual, are evident in the data. These themes can be compared with the typology of suicidal meanings formulated by French historian and sociologist Jean Baechler.[17] When Baechler's typology is used to analyze the data, themes having to do with illness and disability are of particular interest, as are the effects of gender.

Drawing on historical accounts and cross-cultural descriptions of suicide, and using Weber's concept of ideal types, Baechler distinguished eleven types of suicidal meanings, which he grouped together in four categories: escapist, aggressive, oblative, and ludic. In the escapist category, the general meaning or sense of the act is to escape from something or some situation. This general category includes three subtypes: (1) flight, which involves the escape from a general situation sensed by the subject to be intolerable; (2) grief, in which the individual takes his or her life following the loss of a precise and identifiable central element of the personality or way of life; and (3) punishment, in which the act is intended to atone for a real or imagined fault.

The individual committing aggressive suicide seeks to harm someone else. There are four subtypes under this general category of meaning: (1) vengeance, intended either to provoke remorse in someone or to inflict the opprobrium of the community on some person; (2) criminal suicide, in which the individual commits murder and then kills himself or herself, or kills another in order to be killed, or is killed along with other people; (3) blackmail, in which the intent is to put pressure on another person by depriving him or her of something valued; and (4) appeal, in which an individual, by the very nature of the suicide act, is trying to signal that he or she is in danger.

The oblative type of suicide has two subtypes: sacrifice, or the giving up of one's life in order to save or to gain a value judged to be greater, and transfiguration, which seeks to attain a state considered by the individual to be infinitely more delightful than life.

Ludic suicide, the fourth general category in Baechler's classification, finds meaning in either the ordeal or the game. In the ordeal, one risks one's life in order to prove oneself to oneself or to solicit the judgment of others. The game is to take a chance on killing oneself when the sole purpose is to play with one's own life.

I identified several of Baechler's types in the 110 suicides that took place in White Pine County from 1950 to 1990. In terms of gender, there was a vast differential: only 9 of the 110 suicides were women, and they ranged in age from thirteen to seventy. Although 69 percent of the 110 suicides were committed using a firearm, only four of the nine women chose that method. The others used drugs or poison or cut their wrists. Three women left suicide notes.

All of the suicides by women appear to fall under Baechler's general category of escapist suicide, in the subcategories of flight and grief because of the loss of a significant other or the loss of physical integrity. One young girl, for example, had mourned her mother's death for several years and was in conflict with her stepmother. One woman, age thirty-five, left a note to her husband, who had divorced her a few days earlier:

> Remember this, you were my life so I no longer need life itself without you. My wedding ring stays on.[18]

According to the available data, only three of the nine women had physical health problems—one had epilepsy with depression, one had insulin-dependent diabetes, and one suffered from cancer. Although she left no note to confirm it, only the woman with cancer seems to have committed suicide over the state of her health. She had undergone surgery for her cancer some eighteen months before her suicide and had since suffered emotional distress.

When the data available for the 101 males, including twenty-three suicide notes, are analyzed, two of Baechler's four general categories of meaning and three of his subtypes stand out. Escapist suicide was the major category. As was the case with the women, flight and grief due to loss of a significant other or physical integrity were the notable subtypes. However, the general category of aggressive suicide, with criminal suicide as the subtype, was also identified with some of the males; for example, there were four cases in which the man killed his wife or girlfriend and then turned the gun on himself.

In twenty-one cases escapist suicide appeared to be linked with some type of illness or generally poor health. Several of the suicide notes expressed this theme.

A man, age sixty-eight, whose wife had died a few months earlier, left a note to his grandson:

> I've been having chest pains for four or five days and pains over all my body. The doctor told me that I wasn't going to live very long. I know there is a way out [of] this.[19]

Another man left two notes. In one addressed to "the authorities" he said:

> At my age, 69+, I have no desire to go through the hell of a scheduled bowel cancer surgery or the prolonged projected surgeries and the treatments which would likely leave me an invalid. I have no desire to be a burden on someone, especially my wife.

To his wife, he said:

> It has always been my hope that when [the] time came I would go fast, say with a heart attack like my dad or something like that. I would never want to be an invalid or a burden on anyone.[20]

A third man, widowed, age eighty-six, in a note to his son-in-law said:

I can feel myself slipping pretty fast these days. I'm very much afraid of a stroke. My left hand and leg are no good. I have been thinking of this for some time.[21]

In the twenty-one cases in which suicide of males seemed to be linked with illness, a number of factors stand out from the data. First, the diagnosis of cancer, or fear of cancer, was most often mentioned in the suicide context, along with just generally poor health. Second, several individuals spoke of experiencing severe physical pain for various reasons, often over a long period. Third, there seemed to be more fear of *becoming* disabled than of actually *being* disabled, or a least severely disabled.

In the preceding discussion my intent was to present a glimpse of suicide as both a sociological and a psychological phenomenon. But suicide is also a cultural construct. That is, the cultural matrix within which it occurs strongly influences the form, meaning, and frequency of the event. Few investigators have examined the impact and influence of culture on suicide in the United States, because cultural heterogeneity makes such an endeavor extremely difficult. The same is true for a number of other countries, but an attempt was made to address the issue of cultural factors in suicide in nine countries at the Sixth International Congress of the International Association for Suicide Prevention in Mexico City in 1971. Following the presentation of short papers, a list of eight questions was drawn up to serve as a guide for the longer, published versions of the papers:

1. What has been the historical cultural attitude toward suicide?
2. How has the cultural background influenced the form and frequency of suicide?
3. What has been the influence of geography and climate and of religion on the phenomenon?
4. Within the culture, what is the general attitude toward the act today?
5. What is the general attitude toward the person who has committed or attempted suicide?
6. What is the attitude toward the survivors?
7. What are the burial and mourning practices for a suicide?
8. What reflections on suicide are found in the literature, folk songs, art, etc.?[22]

While I do not address each of these questions separately in my discussion of White Pine County, I do use them to frame my discussion. As I have already pointed out, Nevada has a long history of suicide, yet it takes some digging to substantiate this as fact. With so little attention given to the issue by state administrators, the professional literature, and the popular press, the state's cultural attitude toward suicide is best described as indifferent. In contrast, the historical and current attitudes toward suicide in White Pine County are best described as tolerant, if not outright accepting. Even those who express a religious or moral point of view rarely condemn suicide. People's willingness to talk about suicide—both within the family and within the community—makes it apparent that little to no shame or guilt is attached to the act.

Certain concepts identified by Kathleen Ann Long and Clarann Weinert as useful for understanding rural health needs and nursing practices are also helpful in explaining how cultural background influences the form and frequency of suicide.[23] Taking an anthropological, ethnographic approach in their study of rural areas in Montana, Long and Weinert identified the following concepts: work beliefs and health beliefs, isolation and distance, self-reliance, lack of anonymity, outsider/insider, and old-timer/newcomer.

Long and Weinert suggest that in rural populations, work beliefs and health beliefs are closely interrelated in that health is assessed in relation to work role and work activities; health needs are usually secondary to work needs. An excerpt from the suicide note of a fifty-five-year-old Nevada rancher makes this relationship apparent and reveals the importance of the ideal of self-reliance:

> I am a cripple, sick, and dead weight. I do not want to be a load on anyone.
> I have killed a bunch of old dogs and horses to put them out of their misery.
> There is no use fooling myself. I am a worn out has-been. I can not hold a
> job. Bury me as cheap as you can.[24]

The idea of "putting down" old, sick, and hurt animals is very much a part of ranching culture and may carry over into an ideology of suicide that gives a particular cognitive meaning to the act: it is acceptable to "put oneself down" if one is sick and unable to work. This meaning, perhaps embedded in ranching culture, has yet to be fully explored, but it needs to be examined for what it can tell us about suicide in the rural context.

Other aspects of the cultural background that influence suicide in White Pine County are the gun and hunting cultures. The gun culture is reflected in the strong ideology of the "right to bear arms" and in the fact that almost every household owns at least one gun. Given the easy accessibility, it is thus not surprising that firearms are used more frequently for committing suicide than any other means. Hunting for sport and recreation is a major pastime, especially among males. Although it too has not been fully explored, there may be a particular cognitive orientation common to ranching culture and hunting culture regarding the killing of animals and killing in general that fits with an ideology of suicide. This, at least, is the idea inferred in Dayton Duncan's book *Miles from*

Nowhere: Tales from America's Contemporary Frontier. The director of the local mental health center in John Day, Oregon, told Duncan that "killing things . . . isn't that difficult for a population of ranchers, loggers, and hunters. It's what a lot of people do for their income and food. . . . Everybody has a gun and knows how it works. It's [suicide] like hunting; it's no big deal, it's just death."[25]

Duncan discusses another topic relevant to the cultural construction of suicide as well—the boom-and-bust cycles of mining. Again, we know little about the culture of contemporary mining, but by its nature mining is a "close up and move on" enterprise. Duncan suggests that "if the strike is located in a place where there is little else to sustain a concentration of people, the bust is that much more complete. Gold and silver are those kinds of metals. Nevada and Death Valley are those kinds of places."[26] The built-in uncertainty and risk associated with mining fit well with the concept of self-reliance. And when self-reliance can no longer be maintained, for whatever reason, the mining ideology of "closing down and moving on" may be extended to the person in the act of suicide.

Self-reliance may be an aspect of human culture in general rather than merely a part of rural culture and particular subcultures. Some typologies proposed for classifying diverse cultures distinguish between collectivistic and individualistic cultures. Collectivistic cultures are oriented "toward preserving in-group solidarity, even at the expense of placing some limitations on individual expressiveness."[27] In these cultures, suicide disrupts the family and the community's solidarity in the eyes of the larger society, and thus resentment and depreciation of suicidal individuals are to be expected.

Individualistic cultures show a tendency to rely less on the family and more on personal and public sources of relief. "The result may be that individual acts of suicide are less threatening and so less strongly depreciated."[28] The literature on Nevada supports the idea that Nevada prides itself on being and supporting an individualistic cultural orientation. This particular orientation may help to explain the apparent indifference toward suicide.

The question of geography as an influence on suicide in White Pine County relates in part to the concepts of isolation and distance. Even though some residents are amused by *Life* magazine's claim that the "loneliest road in America" leads to Ely, there is a sense of isolation as well in the community, expressed by continual concerns with cutbacks in the intercity bus and airline schedules, and particularly in emergency medical transportation. A coroner's report of the suicide of a lone sheepherder in a distant sheep camp because of pain from a perforated ulcer makes the issue of geography stand out.

White Pine County is a "face-to-face" community in that nearly everyone knows everyone else, or at least knows who the strangers are and why they are there. This general lack of anonymity can also be an aspect of the cultural construction of rural suicide, especially as it relates to mental stress. There is always a shortage of trained mental health professionals in rural Nevada, but even if this were not a problem, many residents of White Pine County would not seek counseling because of the difficulty in maintaining privacy. A sentiment often heard in regard to using the mental health facility is that "people don't want other people to know their business."

Long and Weinert's concepts of insider/outsider and old-timer/newcomer can also be figured into the suicide equation. An often expressed sentiment is that professionals in the community are not very good or well trained or "they wouldn't be in Ely." In other words, there is a general feeling that neither effective mental health services nor adequate medical treatment is available, because "only those that can't practice or make it elsewhere come to Ely." A mental health professional who had been a resident of the county for six or seven years and had young teenage children said that the community would probably not consider his family "insiders" until his future grandchildren grew up.

Although my analysis has focused on an archetypical suicide candidate—a middle-aged or older Caucasian male employed in mining or ranching—two other at-risk groups should be mentioned as well. Three inmates of the maximum security prison in White Pine County have committed suicide since the prison opened in 1990. Thus, the prison not only increased the county's population but also added to the county's suicide statistics. "Prison culture" is now part of the community's diversity and must be included as such. In addition to inmates, there has been an influx of correctional officers—mostly males— from outside the community, some of whom have left their families behind. These individuals, along with the inmates, may be vulnerable to suicide as part of the unique prison culture or as part of the county's rural culture.

Also among the 110 suicides in White Pine County between 1950 and 1990 were three Western Shoshone. The Shoshone pattern of suicide is complex but is often characterized by unemployment and other economic problems.[29] This appeared to be a factor when a Shoshone male committed suicide after learning that he had been rejected for a particular job. However, the pattern of Shoshone suicide identified in the literature warrants further study because of the cultural variation among Shoshone subgroups (e.g., the Western, Eastern, and Northern Shoshone) as well as among rural and urban Shoshone.

Nevada's economy, especially the gains and losses of gaming, is popularly perceived to be the essential cause of the state's high suicide rate. An association between suicide and the economics of mining, with its inherent boom-and-bust cycles, is suggested by the data from White Pine County, as well as by data from Goldfield, Nevada, for the early 1900s.[30] Such economic explanations and associations are tenuous, but they point toward other questions and areas of inquiry. For example, are there underlying cultural constructs shared by the mining and gaming microcultures, and by the microculture of ranching, that support an ideology of suicide? In other words, are there patterns in the cultural scripting of three of Nevada's dominant economies that may help to explain the state's high suicide rate?

One underlying pattern in the microcultures of these economies may be based on the concept of risk. That is, gaming, mining, and to a certain extent ranching in rural Nevada are risk-taking endeavors. This idea of risk taking and suicide was explored by anthropologist Raymond Firth in his studies among the people of Tikopia in Melanesia. Firth argues, for example, that a distinct element of risk taking is involved in the suicide attempts of Tikopians and that risk taking may be built into the structure of ideas about suicide and "may then have a bearing on the sociological interpretation of the volume of suicide."[31] This is an idea worth exploring further in the context of Nevada.

In addition, some of the concepts identified by Long and Weinert for understanding rural health needs may be applicable to the urban context in Nevada.[32] What I am suggesting here is that concepts such as isolation, self-reliance, outsider/insider, and old-timer/newcomer, as well as the concept of individuality, may also be infused into the urban context so as to help construct an ideology of suicide there as well. These concepts may or may not be connected to the urban culture of gaming, and they may or may not inform the cultural scripting of Nevada's long-term urban dwellers as compared with urban newcomers. Again, further research is needed to illuminate the similarities and differences between the urban and rural contexts of suicide.

Nevada is a cultural mosaic, but we ought to search for patterns in this mosaic that tell us more than what can be quantified in statistics or inferred from mental states. We need to know how Nevada fits into the cultural mosaic of the mountain West, with its exceptionally high suicide rate and its large number of places that are "miles from nowhere." If we do not know the cultural makeup of such places, we cannot give meaning to the high numbers. My analysis of White Pine County and Long and Weinert's Montana study suggest that suicides in these regions are at least partly influenced by cultural factors that result from both the environment and the areas' historical socioeconomic basis in ranching and mining. It may be that lives of isolation and individualism, an ethic of self-reliance, and a practical if fatalistic attitude toward death have created a culture in which suicide is viewed as an accepted alternative to life under untenable conditions.

4　White Father Medicine and the Blackfeet, 1855–1955

Native American Health and the Department of the Interior

DIANE D. EDWARDS

In the Blackfeet tradition, sickness and death came to Earth only after Creator Sun saw that humans needed to learn compassion. Because of the suffering that followed, Sun also taught humans about medicinal plants and healing songs, ceremonies, and visions. If such curative efforts failed, the soul of the deceased departed for the Sand Hills, near the present border between Montana and Alberta. This essay centers on that region and on the health care provided to Native Americans there by the U.S. Department of the Interior between 1855 and 1955—health care that, I argue, often reflected a distant bureaucracy incapable or unwilling to respond appropriately to local needs. With an emphasis on nonnative medical practices and a frequently heavy-handed paternalism, the Interior Department nurtured a Native American health care system that might be called "white father medicine."

Despite the system's obvious catastrophic impact on various tribes, few historians have ventured into this particular area of study. Nevertheless, a study of Native American health care in this northernmost part of the mountain West enriches the history of both medicine and public health, and sheds valuable light on important regional issues as well. Here, physical, political, and cultural forces collided as the Interior Department dealt with its Indian wards. A definitive look at this collision would demand comparative studies of separate tribes and regions. Instead I will focus on a smaller area, Blackfeet Agency in Montana, to examine federally funded Native American health care up to 1955 (at which time Indian health services shifted to the Department of Health,

Education, and Welfare). The successes, failures, and frustrations of medical personnel and programs found in this local case study both parallel and reflect the national policy.[1]

Accidents, disease, and war killed Native Americans prior to their extensive contact with Europeans. In the 1820s, cyclic starvation among the still relatively isolated tribes west of the Mississippi River caused conditions "the most pitiable that can be imagined." Nevertheless, the well-being of these people often worsened considerably with their increasing exposure to traders, explorers, and settlers. The reservations created in the late nineteenth century were not only "shrinking islands dirty with lies and greed," as one eyewitness reportedly described them, but crowded with hunger and poverty as well. The concerns of a federal agent for the southern Apaches typified conditions: "They are naked; how am I to clothe them? They want blankets; where and how am I to get them? They have nothing to live on save the stinted ration I have given them, which is not sufficient to feed half the Indians under my charge." Despite widespread recognition that Native Americans' health was in peril, remedial efforts throughout the nineteenth century were both sporadic and inadequate.[2]

The first federal agency accountable for Indian health was the Department of War, which contained an office of Indian affairs from its inception in 1824. An antismallpox program instituted in 1832 was the only organized attempt to protect Native American health during the War Department years. Contract physicians inoculated approximately three thousand native residents along the lower Missouri River. Some tribes refused to participate, and others simply were not included before the $12,000 that funded the project ran out. When the smallpox virus returned in 1837, carried in on steamboats, many thousands died. In the present-day Dakotas and Montana, the Mandan dwindled from 1,600 to 31, and an estimated two-thirds to three-fourths of the Blackfeet peoples perished.[3]

When the Indian Service moved in 1849 to the newly created Department of the Interior, health care again fell victim to the more pressing priorities of settling disputes, gaining access to native lands, and, later, absorbing the Indian into white culture. Much of the nonnative health care came from military physicians and missionaries. For much of the nineteenth century, the federal government subsidized religious groups whose missionary endeavors discouraged or prohibited native healing practices. Little else was attempted by the government until the 1870s, when East Coast reformers began to dominate federal Indian policy. By that time, Native Americans were considered the "vanishing race," and appalling reports of their mistreatment were being published. One plea for reform observed that "all wild Indians, for a period after the process of civilization begins, diminish in numbers. The use of the white man's food, the restraint from roaming, and the ill-ventilated huts in which they dwell, increases diseases, and checks for the time being procreation." The government's solution was threefold: education, Christianity, and agriculture. If the Indian could be turned into an educated Christian farmer, he surely would be a good and happy citizen of the United States.[4]

Medical care and other health concerns rarely emerged as an explicitly stated part of this civilization program before the twentieth century. Although the Interior Department created the Medical and Educational Division in 1873, in practice education remained paramount. Most recipients of federal health care during the late nineteenth century were students at off-reservation boarding schools created to de-Indianize the Indian. But surveys of student and adult health in 1904 finally prompted the department to admit officially that "the Indian, while being fitted for citizenship, is absorbing . . . weakness as well as strength . . . especially true in relation to his physical well-being." Although the department placed the principal blame on the recalcitrant and ignorant Indians themselves, it now felt that "the physical welfare of the Indian is, always must be, the fundamental consideration in any scheme to educate or civilize him. . . . The Indian is worthy the effort to save him, and at the same time it will assist the surrounding whites in removing so many 'plague spots.'" Not until 1924, however, did the Indian Service reorganize and separate its medical and educational services.[5]

Conditions at Blackfeet Agency

The Blackfoot Confederacy consisted of three branches: the Blackfoot, the Bloods, and the Piegans—the North Piegans, in Alberta, and the South Piegans, who live today just east of Glacier National Park on the Blackfeet Reservation. (Hereafter the Piegans of Montana are referred to as Blackfeet, in line with contemporary sources.) When the United States made its first treaty with the Blackfeet in 1855, all traveled freely between what is now southern Montana and central Alberta. The treaty greatly reduced the size of Blackfeet territory and established an agency in what is now north-central Montana. Agency officials were responsible for about 5,800 Blackfoot, Bloods, and Piegans, as well as 2,600 of their allies, the Gros Ventres.

Each tribe was to have a physician and a hospital, but medical treatment remained meager long after the treaty was signed. At least through 1863, lists of required supplies did not include medicines or physician salaries, even though government agents remarked on the "pinching hunger and chilling cold" among an Indian nation they called "farther off from civilization than any tribes on the Missouri River." Local agents had to rely on temporary physicians and emergency medical supplies to treat their wards. As elsewhere in the nation, little was done specifically to improve health on the reservation before the

1870s. By that time four smallpox epidemics had considerably weakened a tribe once considered one of the fiercest in the West. Smallpox among a Piegan band attacked in 1870 by unprovoked U.S. Army troops not only helped the army to victory but was concealed in the official report to Washington, prompting public outrage when it was finally exposed.[6]

In the last decades of the nineteenth century, the Blackfeet needed a decent food supply far more than they needed white physicians or their medicines. Interested whites, particularly in the distant East, clung to an image of the Blackfeet as a healthy, noble warrior society of "wild, dusky men [who] sweep like a whirlwind over the arid deserts of the central plateau." In reality, the bison herds had vanished from Montana by 1882 and the government rations were not enough for the 3,209 enrolled at the agency. During the summer of 1883, an inspector investigating charges of fraud at the agency found less than one-fourth of the flour needed for the upcoming winter and less than one-fifth of the standard beef ration. A Senate subcommittee that visited in September concluded that the Blackfeet and their allies, compared with more prosperous tribes in the area, were "in wretched condition, and their future almost hopeless . . . it was pitiable to see the eagerness in the hungry eyes of the waiting crowd as the beef was being distributed." Despite orders from the Washington office to increase weekly rations until the following May, an estimated one quarter of the U.S. Blackfeet died during the so-called Starvation Winter of 1883–84.[7]

By the twentieth century, food was more plentiful but health and living conditions remained substandard. Despite a low tuberculosis rate relative to those of many other tribes surveyed in 1904, in general the Blackfeet shared the high incidence of diseases found throughout the native West. A 1912 U.S. Public Health Service (PHS) study found the overall nationwide death rate among Indians to be three times that for the white population. Twenty-six percent of those examined in Montana had trachoma, a serious eye infection that could cause blindness. The inspector assigned to the Blackfeet reservation attributed the high rate of disease to "filthy habits, insanitary homes, and the use of intoxicants." Any curative medical efforts, said the PHS report, were "largely nullified by the conditions under which the [physicians'] work is attempted and by the indifference of the primitive Indian and his ignorance of the first principles of hygienic living."[8]

As early as 1889 the Interior Department had recognized the importance of preventive medicine, instructing its physicians to attend to sanitation and its field matrons to help raise living standards in homes. Nevertheless, years passed before comprehensive sanitation and other preventive programs became standard policy. When inspector Elsie Newton assessed Blackfeet Agency and the nearby town of Browning in 1914, she criticized the latter's principal source of water, open creeks bordered by pit privies. The reservation itself was "a few de-

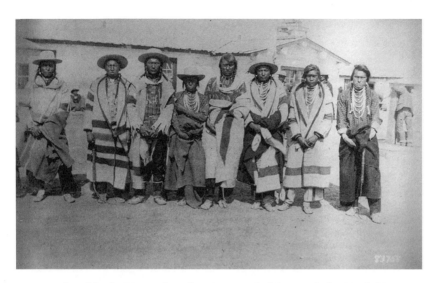

By 1889, when this photo was taken, the Montana Blackfeet regularly visited the agency headquarters on ration day to receive what they believed were inadequate supplies of beef, flour, beans, and coffee. Courtesy National Archives, photo no. 111-SC-83758.

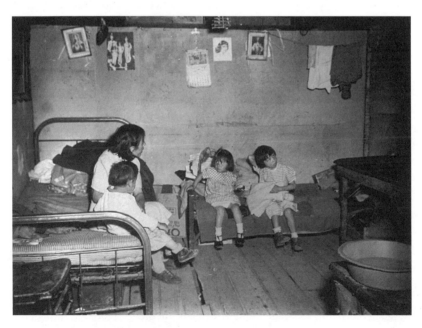

When federal inspectors visited the Blackfeet reservation in 1951, they found that residents still lived in inadequate housing such as this home of several Cut Bank Boarding School students. Courtesy National Archives, photo no. RG75-N-660.

grees better than on some reservations and many degrees better than on others [due to less refuse around homes] . . . comparable to the average rural home." Two years later the Indian office reported that a particularly aggressive house-to-house cleanup in the Heart Butte area of the reservation had permanently re-solved the environmental problems. Subsequently, fifty households on the reservation received a form letter from Washington exhorting recipients to fol-low "nature's laws of cleanliness and right-living, which we must all obey if we wish to be well and happy."[9]

But poor conditions persisted in the Heart Butte district, home to most of the 1,200-plus full-bloods, despite the cleanup campaign. Just before World War I, 90 percent of the district's residents were reported to have trachoma, and perhaps 75 percent had tuberculosis. Various surveys claimed that the reserva-tion as a whole had a trachoma rate of 60–75 percent and a tuberculosis rate of 50–75 percent. Clifton Rosin, the physician treating the full-bloods, warned the Washington office: "Unless something substantial, something adequate is done for their welfare . . . what is the use of planning for their future welfare, for with-out the tenant, we will have no need for the house."[10]

The house improved very little during the 1920s, admittedly difficult years throughout rural America. An exhaustive study of reservations by the National Tuberculosis Association blamed the high incidence of tuberculosis, trachoma, and other diseases during the 1910s and early 1920s on unhealthy environments (and skimpy budgets). As a group, the Blackfeet were neither the worst nor the best in terms of tuberculosis morbidity and mortality. But following a visit in 1920, Hugh Scott, a member of the independent Board of Indian Commission-ers, called Blackfeet Agency "one of the most neglected and run-down places in the Indian Service." When Scott returned in 1924, he found agency superin-tendent Fred Campbell in charge of "the most encouraging of all the Indian agencies I have visited." Two things, according to Scott, had made the differ-ence: Campbell's five-year economic plan to encourage self-sufficiency and the agency's method of treating trachoma.[11]

The actual conditions were far more bleak than Scott's report implied. In 1928 an influential report from the Institute for Government Research again ex-coriated the Interior Department for its dealings with its Indian wards, includ-ing the continued lack of adequate preventive measures. Of paramount impor-tance were the unhealthful conditions on reservations like that of the Blackfeet, where a recent meningitis outbreak had overtaxed health services. Visitors in the 1930s got the same visual "knockout blow on the chin," according to agency physician Herman F. Schrader. One visitor commented, "It looks as though the children of Lazarus had squatted here." Anxious for health care, the Blackfeet appealed not only to local officials but also to the Indian Service's Washington office, the president, and the public. One sent form letters to chambers of commerce across the country, asking for clothing, bedding, and soap. By June 1937, ration supplies for the old and indigent were exhausted. When a request for additional money was denied, a resident—one-eighth Blackfeet and labeled a troublemaker by the superintendent—wrote to Montana senator Burton K. Wheeler for help because conditions were "not as they should be and the outlook for the coming winter is gloomy and sad." [12]

After the Depression, World War II again diverted both official attention and government funds from the reservations. The military drained physicians from the already understaffed Indian Service. Blackfeet Agency was down to two physicians when, in 1941, Superintendent Roy Nash sent a memo to the tribal council, farm agents, reservation priests, and others. If possible, he advised, patients should be brought to the hospital rather than relying on field services. At the same time, the agency was serving more patients than any other reservation in the state. In a recent year, the medical staff had made more than three thousand house calls, held thirteen clinics, scheduled three thousand office calls, and driven nearly forty thousand miles to treat 4,700 cases within the one-million-acre reservation. The field nurse had a caseload of nearly five hundred children, many with trachoma, and the new forty-five-bed hospital was one of the busiest of its size in the Indian Service. Still, problems persisted with dental disease, trachoma, venereal disease, infant mortality, and tuberculosis, the last accounting for one-third of the recorded deaths. [13]

The end of World War II brought little relief to the Blackfeet. When Medical Officer Warren R. Creviston visited the agency in March and April 1947, there was only one physician on-site when there should have been three, and only one field nurse. Tuberculosis had killed seventy-five people during the previous year, there was very little follow-up on surviving cases, and the number of trachoma cases was also high. For the remainder of the decade, Blackfeet Agency's health services limped along understaffed, underfunded, and unnoticed. Then, in the particularly severe winter of 1949–50, with roads impassable and temperatures below zero, an Associated Press story appeared nationwide reporting that the Blackfeet were "eating skunk and porcupine to fight off starvation." This time it was the public that demanded immediate government and presidential action. [14]

Federal Authority, Local Activity

In 1880 there were seventy-seven full- and part-time physicians in the Indian Service, serving more than 200,000 potential patients. Policy changes within the Interior Department during the next three decades would suggest a real commitment to Indian medical services, and it might seem that Indian health, including that of the Blackfeet, was finally on the road to recovery. Nurses and field matrons joined Indian Service ranks, although they worked almost exclusively at the boarding schools. Official interest shifted somewhat from education and civilization toward health and living conditions. In its 1904 annual report, the Interior Department asserted that "greater stress has been laid upon questions affecting the health of Indians, both in and out of school, than heretofore." Reflecting this change in attitude, the department appointed a chief medical supervisor in 1909, putting Indian health for the first time under professional medical supervision. Two years later, Congress authorized $40,000 for *general* health services for Indians, the first such allocation.[15]

But a national budget and policy did not ensure effective action for individual reservations. President William H. Taft noted the high tuberculosis rate among the Blackfeet in his 1912 call to Congress for improved medical care capable of giving the Indian race "a physically efficient maturity." But health care was just one of many problems at Blackfeet Agency, and often not the first priority. In his reports to Washington, Superintendent Fred Campbell vacillated between two primary goals for his wards—teaching them a trade and keeping them healthy. In 1924 he wrote that "it doubtless goes without saying that the health situation is the important feature on our Indian reservation, and even takes precedence to the industrial features." A year later, however, Campbell objected to a plan to replace his three field matrons with trained nurses, an opinion lamented by the Indian Service's public health nursing supervisor after her visit to the agency. Campbell was a man who believed in "health through industry," and his field matrons were teaching self-sufficiency, a goal more important than health. "I do not think," he wrote, that "there is any other tribe of people in the world that run to the doctor and nurses as do the Indian people, much of which could be remedied by their own industrial efforts if they could only be brought to see it."[16]

Despite Campbell's pride in his economic program, it was the agency's efforts to fight trachoma that attracted national attention. The disease had long been a problem on the reservations, despite an antitrachoma campaign initiated by the federal government in 1911. In the 1920s physicians suspected that an unidentified microorganism caused the potentially blinding disease. Standard treatments of scrubbing the inside of the eyelid with chemicals or surgically removing growths frequently failed. When a University of Pennsylvania professor of ophthalmology named L. Webster Fox visited Glacier National Park in 1923, he convinced an agency physician to learn his radical tarsectomy method (excision of connective tissue in the eyelid). Fox later held court at the agency, training several Indian Service physicians from the western reservations. Assistant Commissioner E. B. Merrit told Superintendent Campbell that he wanted to showcase the Blackfeet trachoma program as an indication of what might be done on other reservations. Unfortunately for the patients, Fox's method was largely ineffective, and the service was later castigated for blindly accepting and implementing an unproved method. In 1934 an Indian Service ophthalmologist told Superintendent Forrest Stone that doctors were still trying "to overcome some of the bad results" from the Fox clinic. Shortly thereafter, Blackfeet Agency served as one of the service's two pilot sites for another controversial treatment, the pneumothorax procedure for tuberculosis.[17]

Financially overburdened during the 1930s, the Indian Service became more selective about who was qualified to receive its health care, a national-level policy that had local results. The Blackfeet had begun to make specific demands on Washington for more medical services. At least one historian has noted the especially dramatic increase in Blackfeet hospital births during this period. To ameliorate the situation, local officials placed some patients in other government or private facilities both in and outside the state, with varied success. They relayed to the Washington office numerous requests to subsidize health care off the reservation. The commissioner's office, for instance, authorized no more than $240 for one patient's treatment at the Montana State Hospital for the Feeble Minded. It became increasingly difficult to reimburse nonreservation hospitals and physicians treating Blackfeet patients, thus straining relations with outside institutions such as the Stanford University School of Medicine and with private physicians and hospitals in neighboring towns. Blanch Fuller, the superintendent of Montana Deaconess Hospital in Great Falls, wrote President Franklin D. Roosevelt directly to complain that her institution had not been reimbursed by the agency for several years' service to the amount of $3,652. Problems arose with other agencies too, as Blackfeet traveled to other reservations in the state for medical care.[18]

Especially vexing was the placement of adult tuberculosis patients and the retention of juvenile patients. One tribal member asked that her twenty-four-year-old son be sent to the service's Lapwai Sanatorium in Idaho, a request denied because the facility admitted only school-age children. "All I can manage to do," she wrote, "is made [*sic*] a living, and if he can get a patent to his land he can pay for his care afterwards, but something must be done for him at once, and I demand help for him." This case undercuts the claim made by Superintendent Stone that "if in any way the Indian as a race have [*sic*] criminal tendencies, I would say that perhaps their greatest crime lies in the indifferent attitude they take towards the proper care of their children." Dr. Schrader, the senior agency physician, had a somewhat different view of why parents refused to place their children in the local tuberculosis sanatorium: "Family ties are very strong among Indians, and they share their poverty to the danger point, which is to their credit, they are helpless and know it, and in this problem of tuberculosis we are almost as helpless and also know it."[19]

As federal funds dwindled, the Interior Department placed even tighter restrictions on eligibility for health services. Acceptable applicants had to be on the Blackfeet tribal rolls and able to prove that they were indigent. The fact that deserving patients were sometimes excluded is shown by the case of Mrs. W., a woman who lived on the reservation. In 1931, she wrote to Stone for authorization to go to a Cardston, Alberta, dentist to have her teeth pulled at a cost of $100 to ease her "continual suffering." Roads to the dentist in nearby Cut Bank were impassable and there was no government dentist available. She would not have asked for money at all, she said, if her husband, who was white, had had a job. Unfortunately, Mrs. W. held a fee patent to a few acres, which she was thus permitted to sell, and the Government Accounting Office had already ruled that gratuity funds could not be used by "Indian" fee-patent holders. Native women married to white men, and therefore considered to be without need, could also be denied assistance.[20]

The health status of the Native American nationwide *had* improved somewhat by the 1930s. The Indian Service's chief medical director, James G. Townsend, told the State and Provincial Health Authorities of North America in 1936 that the Indian death rate had dropped in the past twenty-five years from 35.6 to 15.1 per 1,000. There were seventy-six general Indian Service hospitals and thirteen tuberculosis sanatoria, as well as working relationships with the Public Health Service, the Phipps Institute in Philadelphia, universities, and other federal agencies. But Townsend also admitted that Indian health remained poor compared with that of the white population; for example, tuberculosis mortality among some Indian groups was twenty times that among the white population. It was, Townsend said, a complex and costly situation: "The whole matter [of health] is so bound up in economics, food, recreation, etc., it is difficult to estimate sometimes which is cause and which is effect."[21]

Between 1940 and 1950, the life expectancy of Native Americans increased by nine years, but progress was still slow compared with the health status of the general population. The white population in Montana had one of the lowest infant death rates in the nation, but the rate for the state's Native Americans was more than four times higher, a figure indicative of complex problems that resisted simple solutions. The principal culprit varied according to the accuser. An American Medical Association survey team that visited the Blackfeet placed the primary fault on the Indian Service's inadequate appreciation of its own physicians, whose dedication despite the working conditions took "some kind of missionery [sic] spirit." The Blackfeet reservation at the foot of the Rocky

Mountains stood a long way from the central office in Washington. So did the agency's health care professionals and their medical facilities.[22]

Blackfeet Health Care—Process and Performance

In 1878 the Interior Department attempted to raise health standards on the reservations by employing only graduates of approved medical colleges. The government later placed physicians under civil service regulations, which required them to pass competency exams. The department sought men who were "temperate, industrious, professional, and dedicated" to overcome the influence of native medicine men, teach hygiene, visit schools, and treat in-office patients. What it got was a workforce of uneven competence, often disgruntled by local conditions, the distant central office, the lack of professional recognition, and conflicts with native healers. Most of the health care provided to the Blackfeet was probably the best possible under the prevailing conditions. But for decades, local medical personnel joined reservation residents, the press, reformers, and private health professionals in repeatedly criticizing the Interior Department for its substandard and understaffed facilities.[23]

From the beginning reservation superintendents had seen the value of having physicians as part of their permanent staffs, but medical men were not always an unadulterated blessing. In 1872, Blackfeet Agency got what appears to have been its first full-time physician, Dr. J. C. Sills, who performed admirably during an outbreak of erysipelas. The doctor's tendency toward drunkenness, however, prompted the next agent to request (unsuccessfully) that Dr. Sills's services be replaced by visiting U.S. Army medical officers from Fort Shaw, thirty-five miles away to the southwest. Problems still existed forty years later, when the entire medical staff was dismissed after the superintendent sent photos of their dispensary and personal living quarters, all in filthy disarray, to Washington. When the Washington supervisor arrived to view the situation firsthand, a delegation of Blackfeet was waiting to lodge complaints. Not long afterward, Drs. Rosin and Stauffer were quarreling and Rosin was "mixed up in a liquor scandal." In 1926, the three physicians resident at the agency, graduates of Western University of Canada, Marquette University, and Chicago Homeopathic College, were again a mixed blessing. One was "overbearing, antagonistic, without diplomacy . . . [and] unpopular wherever he has been stationed." Another, a former farmer, had a poor personality, dirty fingernails, and shabby clothes, but was well liked by his patients, according to the district medical director.[24]

Physicians and patients had to overcome more than insufferable personalities and personal conflicts. The conditions for practicing medicine would have hindered even the most determined and dedicated doctor. When physician M. A. Miller first arrived at the agency in October 1884, he wrote to the Washington office, "There are no Library *whatever,* no Instruments, and scarcely any Drugs, and what are here ⅓ should be condemned [*sic*] as they are damaged." He requested approval to purchase eight specific medical texts, syringes, a thermometer, towels and cotton, a stethoscope, and a speculum. Apparently Miller's disgust with the situation remained unremedied. The following summer, agent R. A. Allen wrote to Washington that Miller had just left for his home in Pennsylvania, and that it was "very desirable that another Physician come here as soon as possible." A nearby group of Poplar River Indians had just contracted smallpox, and Blackfeet Agency had neither vaccine nor a physician to treat them.[25]

Although working conditions at Blackfeet Agency gradually improved, they fell far short of those expected or desired. Well into the twentieth century, employee housing at the agency was considered among the worst in the Indian Service, and the Washington-mandated bureaucracy was enough to drive local officials to distraction. In 1918, for instance, Blackfeet Agency sent 15,106 communications and received 10,350, of which 7,230 and 5,450, respectively, were to and from the main office. Physicians often were reprimanded for not submitting adequate and frequent enough reports and for not keeping useful statistics. Salaries were not always paid on time, and government cars for fieldwork were in short supply. Car rationing was a sore point with the field nurses who cared for patients in remote homes. The situation eroded morale among Indian Service personnel. In 1939, one physician at Blackfeet Agency unsuccessfully asked Washington to publish a periodical for and by his peers, to help alleviate "those problems of disinterestedness" among service physicians, men with "truly interesting and valuable original ideas who see the burial of those ideas."[26]

The harsh conditions also imposed physical hardships on health care workers, particularly during the frequent staff shortages, and no doubt influenced the care given to patients. With only one physician and one nurse on the staff during a 1920 influenza outbreak, Superintendent Horace Wilson telegraphed Washington for authority to employ two extra nurses for thirty days. His request denied, he grumbled that it was no wonder friends tried to raise money to take patients to private hospitals elsewhere. Getting enough nurses strained the resources of agency officials, a problem the national office recognized when it created a field matron and public health nurse unit in 1924. Within two years, Blackfeet Agency had a full nursing staff: a graduate nurse, a public school nurse, and a public health nurse on loan from the Montana Tuberculosis Association. Despite Superintendent Campbell's doubts about nurses versus field matrons, the former had secured a place on the reservation. Like the physicians, the nursing staff changed frequently and endured crushing workloads. In 1931, several epidemics contributed to what Superintendent Stone called "a general break down of [nurses'] health" that left the hospital with thirty to forty patients and no nursing staff.[27]

Poor facilities also impeded the efficient delivery of health care. Standing "far out to itself upon a bleak prairie," the hospital-turned-sanatorium constructed in 1915 did not fit the local climate, being built from the same plans used for Indian Service structures in more temperate areas—and without storm windows and doors. Its operation consistently exceeded the $10,000 annual budget, much to the dismay of the Washington office, which wondered why the Blackfeet sanatorium cost more per capita to operate than others in the service. The standard reasons given—more fuel and clothing needed because of cold weather—were not satisfactory, and the local staff had to operate without additional funds. During the Depression tribal members more readily returned to the reservation, and the facilities were inadequate to deal with the added load. Eventually the sanatorium reverted to a general hospital, albeit one poorly equipped and difficult to clean. Workers sterilized surgical materials in a small household pressure cooker and did without a sterilizing dishwasher and a working microscope. An inspector found conditions there "reprehensible."[28]

It no longer sufficed for supervisors to assure their field physicians that low pay and horrid working conditions paled before the noble work of lifting Indians out of "their superstitious regard for the grotesque rites" of medicine men. The equipment was bad, the libraries obsolete, the housing poor, and the chances for postgraduate education nil. Physicians needed permission to mail a letter or make a phone call. Blackfeet Agency physician Theodore Crabbe claimed in 1950 that it took so long to get Washington's authorization for sanatorium hospitalization that the patient often no longer wanted to go. Many physicians, Crabbe said, saw the Indian Service as "a political football of uncertain and indefinite longevity. The last quarter of each fiscal year work is curtailed for fear of running in the red, and first quarter of the new fiscal year money is not available because Congress had not yet voted a new appropriation."[29]

Despite budgetary and personnel shortages during and after World War II, tribal populations nationwide used federal health facilities and services in ever greater numbers. By the 1940s, about 75–80 percent of Native American births occurred in hospitals, compared with 50 percent for the general U.S. population and no more than 10 percent for comparable economic groups. (Birthrates among Native Americans had risen to 35 percent higher than the rate for the general population.) More than one out of every five reservation residents used hospital services, compared with one out of fifteen in the general population. In addition, there were more Native American health workers and greater tribal council involvement in health activities. Despite all this and a decreasing death rate, Native Americans still died at a rate 25 percent greater than that of the general population.[30]

Rhetoric in Washington turned increasingly to termination; that is, to abrogating federal responsibility for all Native American programs. In 1948, a task force on policy concluded that *this* time the solution to the obdurate Indian problem was a transfer of services, especially to state and local agencies. There had been termination talk for decades, but in 1955 Congress took the first step toward the eventual elimination of the Indian Service. Indian health care was moved to the Department of Health, Education, and Welfare (HEW), organizational home to the Public Health Service officers the Interior Department had been utilizing for many years. With it went 3,500 employees, one-fourth of the Bureau of Indian Affairs staff. The transfer of health services was not a new idea: In 1919 the U.S. surgeon general had argued against a similar proposal because medical issues were too tightly tied to the educational, social, and industrial problems of "a race in its critical social and economic transition." Opinion among the Native American population was split over the transfer; the Blackfeet were among those supporting the move, no doubt hoping for improved health care.[31]

Lessons (Un)learned

It is clear from the Blackfeet experience that, despite some successes, the Department of the Interior was a less than exemplary health care provider. When health care services were moved to the HEW in 1955, the 1911 appropriation of $40,000 had grown to an annual budget of more than $40 million. Yet, other than diseases for which there were vaccines and sera, disease prevalence among Native Americans was as high relative to the general population as it had been in 1911. In 1955, the death rate from measles was twenty times the general rate and nine times that from tuberculosis. The tuberculosis rate in 1955 was the same as the general population's rate had been in 1938, and the infant mortality rate was the same as that for all races in 1931—a difference of seventeen and twenty-four years, respectively.

Why wasn't the Interior Department more effective in providing health care for Native Americans? And how did Blackfeet health care compare with that on other reservations, and with that in similar socioeconomic groups, the general population, and the rest of the Blackfoot Confederacy in Alberta, Canada?[32]

The broadest answers to the first question are the most obvious: an obfuscating difficulty in assigning priorities, a shortage of funds for medical services, and a geographic region far removed from the policy makers. In the early nineteenth century, the *control* of the Indian was of utmost concern. Later in the century, education and Christianization diverted resources. By the twentieth century, health-related problems had shifted, intensified, and become more costly. While "scientific medicine" was suppressing some serious diseases such as smallpox, other disorders associated with sanitation and nutrition were increasing. Mention of conditions on the Blackfeet reservation bolstered arguments for programs to combat these new health problems. Two costly world wars and a severe economic depression were partly to blame for the "political parsimony" responsible, some said, and for the continued spread of death and disease among Indians. But physical and cultural isolation likewise contributed. Unlike some tribal groups, the Blackfeet attracted little media attention, were not constituents of eastern politicians or reformers, and did not control large reserves of natural resources. By mid-century, the Indian Service's own medical director complained that too much public notice had been paid to the plight of the Navajo, diverting resources from the equally imperiled Blackfeet. What publicity the latter did receive came largely from visitors to nearby Glacier National Park, created in 1910 partly from lands ceded by the tribe.[33]

Answering the second question—how the health of the Blackfeet compared with that of other groups—is more difficult because comparative studies and studies set within the larger social context are largely nonexistent. Some diseases seem to have affected the Blackfeet and their neighbors more seriously than they affected other Native Americans. In the late 1940s, the tuberculosis death rate among Montana Indians was somewhat less than that for the Navajo, for example, yet the death rate from infantile diarrhea among Blackfeet children was about twice that among Navajo children. Conversely, the Blackfeet infant death rate in general was only half that of the Navajo. Using a comparison closer to home, tribes in Wyoming had a death rate from pneumonia more than three times the tribal rates in Montana. Suggestive as these crude comparisons are, definitive answers must come from closer scrutiny of both tribal and disease diversity. Stephen Kunitz has argued that America's historically nomadic tribes were less adaptable to communal reservation living than were agriculturalist groups, and thus exhibited different disease patterns. Whether or not this holds true for the once-nomadic Blackfeet awaits further study.[34]

The need for comparative research points to a need for more regional studies, as well as for studies that examine factors such as interaction with native healers and health care provided by religious and military organizations. One regional study now under way will compare the health services provided to the Blackfoot of Alberta with those provided to the Blackfeet in Montana, groups nearly identical in their cultural and physical geography. They shared hunting grounds, a language, and, to their detriment, epidemic diseases. Each also at times shared the other's government services, from rations in the nineteenth century to health care as late as 1949. The U.S. and Canadian governments had different approaches to their respective "Indian problems," and reformers and government officials in the United States consistently pointed to the Canadian system as superior. Yet Hana Samek, in her study of the Blackfoot Confederacy to 1920, concluded that the Canadian government basically ignored native health until after World War I, relying instead on religious, philanthropic, and private institutions to provide medical services, and reacted only to emergencies such as epidemics.[35]

During the Interior Department years, health-related conditions on the Montana reservation and the responses of both the Washington office and its local employees coexisted within an unavoidably larger context of politics, culture, and economics, a context in which general apathy and bureaucratic neglect flourished. The various western reservations that sanitary engineer H. Norman Old surveyed in the early 1950s were "nearly half a century in arrears with respect to the application of sanitary science to disease prevention. . . . With the exception of some immunization procedures and limited field nursing services for a few of the tribes, no preventive disease measures or public health educational programs reaching the individual Indian home or community ha[d] been attempted." In 1953, Fred T. Foard, chief of the BIA's health branch, blamed Native Americans' high tuberculosis death rate on "inexcusable health conditions" allowed by public apathy. Shortly before the interagency transfer of health services, Oliver LaFarge wrote: "While white Americans by the thousands enjoy the romance and color of the Indians, and love to sentimentalize about them, they do not give a whoop in hell whether they live well, die in misery, or just drag along in weary, broken despair."[36]

The relief of misery and despair historically stands as the principal purpose of public health programs, whether local or national in scope. Although distinct in its day-to-day details, health care at Blackfeet Agency inevitably reflected decision making at the national level that ranged from virtual neglect to near obsession with cleanliness and social uplift. Patients at the agency responded as patients did elsewhere, incorporating the federally provided services into their own healing and life-style systems. Stephen Kunitz has argued that, at least in recent decades, Indian health has benefited by its separation from local and state jurisdictions. But for Blackfeet Agency caregivers and patients during the period described here, the physical and bureaucratic isolation frustrated both the personnel and the delivery of health care. Concurrently, the nationwide failure to implement sustained preventive programs, long after their importance was recognized, impinged on health vis-à-vis local environmental conditions. With regard to relieving the misery and despair of the Blackfeet of Montana, the federal bureaucracy responsible for shaping native health care policies prior to 1955 seems to have been, despite individual good intentions, unable or unwilling to succeed.

5   The Scientific Construction of New Diseases

Rocky Mountain Spotted Fever and

AIDS as Comparative Case Studies

VICTORIA A. HARDEN

Rocky Mountain spotted fever and acquired immunodeficiency syndrome (AIDS) are diseases that have affected people in the mountain West during the twentieth century. The former was first recognized just before the century began; the latter toward its end. Using these two diseases as case studies, I will examine how twentieth-century medical scientists have constructed infectious diseases as intellectual phenomena and I will ask whether place played a role in their understanding. I will argue that geographical place has more relevance to the social construction of novel twentieth-century diseases than to their scientific construction. I will further contend that a set of shared ideas about disease causation—the germ theory of infectious diseases and a corollary of this theory relating to host immune defenses—informed the scientific construction of both diseases. These assertions run somewhat counter to much recent scholarship on the highly specific localization of scientific fact construction within individual laboratories, and to much social history scholarship as well.[1] Nonetheless, I hope to demonstrate that this single paradigm provided the intellectual framework for understanding both Rocky Mountain spotted fever and AIDS.[2]

Intellectual Framework: The Germ Theory

Before the advent of the germ theory, physicians conceptualized disease as the result of an imbalance in the humors, or body fluids. The disequilibrium might be caused by forces as uncontrollable as the inauspicious alignment of heavenly bodies or by the bad habits or moral defects of individuals. Physicians sought to restore the humoral balance by individualistic prescriptions and also, when appropriate, supported societal repentance and prayers for heavenly interdiction. Toward the end of the nineteenth century, a new paradigm supplanted the humoral approach as an explanation for the causation of infectious diseases. This new intellectual framework asserted that pathologic bacteria and protozoa, known generically as "germs," gained access to human tissues and produced the fevers, rashes, pains, and other manifestations of infectious diseases.[3] The power of this "germ theory" to overturn centuries of traditional medicine lay in its ability to guide effective intervention in the disease process. For example, one corollary of the theory explained how microorganisms were transmitted from host to host. Water contaminated with disease microorganisms was early identified as such a vector, and epidemics could be halted dramatically if water supplies were kept free of the body fluids of diseased people. This was compelling evidence that the germ theory reflected biological reality. During ensuing decades, additional pathogenic microorganisms were identified, including a submicroscopic class called viruses.

Additional discoveries throughout the twentieth century—especially the development of antibiotics that could cure bacterial infections—further buttressed the new paradigm. In the 1970s, another corollary of the germ theory, one dealing with how human hosts defend themselves against invading microorganisms, became an extremely fruitful field of inquiry. After many decades of unsatisfactory speculation, sophisticated techniques at last illuminated the relationship between the humoral and cellular components of the immune system. The lymphocytes of the blood were found to be subdivided into T (thymus-derived) cells and B (bone marrow–derived) cells, and the major functions performed by each type were described. Histocompatibility complexes, which helped other immune system components distinguish self from nonself, were identified. Substances called cytokines were recognized as mediators of the immune processes. As the twentieth century entered its last two decades, the details of this germ theory corollary were being studied intensely for potential disease-intervention strategies.[4]

Rocky Mountain Spotted Fever

It is difficult to examine the influence of the germ theory on the construction of infectious diseases because the theory itself is now so widely accepted that infectious diseases are defined within its constructs. Rocky Mountain spotted fever, for example, is described as one of the so-called diseases of nature, which normally exist "silently" in the natural world and affect human beings only when they intrude into the habitats of the causative microorganisms. *Dermacentor andersoni,* the Rocky Mountain wood tick, was the first spotted fever vector identified. The female tick transmits the pathogenic organism, *Rickettsia rickettsii,* to the next generation in her eggs. The disease organisms are tiny bacteria that, like viruses, must inhabit living cells to metabolize and reproduce.[5] The definition of spotted fever given here specifies the disease as the physiological manifestations of infection with the causative agent.

A similar understanding of the infectious process explains the progression of signs and symptoms that characterize the disease in humans. Between three days and two weeks after being bitten by an infected tick, the victim suffers a splitting headache and a fever that may rise to 104° F. The characteristic spots of the disease appear first on the wrists and ankles, then spread to cover the entire body, including the palms of the hands and the soles of the feet. Few diseases generate rashes that appear on the palms and soles, hence this sign is usually considered diagnostic in conjunction with high fever and history of tick bite. In fulminant cases of the disease, the patient may die before the spots appear. Some of those who recover experience severe neurological sequelae. Within the accepted twentieth-century understanding of Rocky Mountain spotted fever, all of these symptoms are linked to the action of rickettsial organisms. Once they have gained access to the patient's body via the bite of an infected tick, the rickettsiae attack the endothelial cells in the capillaries of the circulatory tree. As these cells swell and burst, the capillaries become permeable, resulting, in about 20 percent of cases, in circulatory collapse and death. Blood leaking through into the skin causes the spots that accompany the fever. This rash is a palpable purpura—that is, it can be felt under the skin even though it appears flat. The neurological symptoms and sequelae are not as well understood but are similarly linked to rickettsial attack on capillaries in the brain.[6]

Geographically, Rocky Mountain spotted fever is limited to the Western Hemisphere, and is further limited to particular areas that are ecologically suitable habitats for the vector tick. The disease was first identified in the Rocky Mountain region of North America, hence its name. That name led to its description by one early investigator as a "place disease, being definitely limited to a certain locality." By the end of the nineteenth century the disease was well known throughout the Northwest in localized areas.[7] In the Snake River valley of Idaho, for example, a mild form of the disease with a low mortality was widely recognized. In 1896, the first published report on the disease appeared, in the annual report of Major Marshall W. Wood, a U.S. Army physician stationed in Boise, Idaho. In 1899, an Idaho physician named Edward E. Maxey, the secretary of the Idaho State Medical Society, published the first paper on spotted fever in a medical journal.[8]

In Colorado and Oregon, spotted fever was described as having "considerable mortality" and was reported most frequently in the foothills in the central part of eastern Oregon. No case was known west of the Cascade Mountains.[9] In Wyoming, spotted fever apparently had been known by travelers on the Oregon Trail, who called it mountain typhus, mountain sickness, mountain fever, and trail typhus. The disease plagued them particularly from "the point where the trail joined the Sweetwater River about at Independence Rock" until they crossed the Green River. This description coincides with the central and north-central location of the majority of Wyoming cases.[10] Other investigators have concluded that spotted fever was also present in Washington, Nevada, Utah, and California when Europeans arrived.[11]

An especially virulent strain of the disease occurred in the Bitterroot Valley of Montana, and this is where research on the disease began. Spotted fever apparently emerged in this location when white settlers, most of whom arrived after the Civil War, disrupted the ecology of the valley.[12] Extensive lumbering operations driven by the construction of railroads drastically reduced the forests on the west side of the valley. The trees were replaced by scrub vegetation, ideal habitat for wood ticks. Even though less than 5 percent of the ticks were infected with the organism that causes spotted fever, they were sufficient to transmit the disease each spring to a dozen or so of the people who ventured into the scrublands and canyons on the west side of the valley.[13]

The earliest medical perceptions of spotted fever did not connect lumbering activities with spotted fever. They reflected instead the medical community's awareness—if not complete acceptance—of the newly proposed germ theory. Because the disease was often contracted during the spring by people who traveled in mountain canyons and drank melted snow, some physicians conversant with the concept of water as a disease vector speculated that spotted fever might be waterborne, like cholera or typhoid fever. Others, observing that the disease might strike only one member of a group who had drunk from a common water supply, fell back on older concepts of miasmas rising from the earth as the cause.[14]

From the beginning of official inquiry, however, scientific investigators were solidly grounded in the germ theory of disease, and none gave credence to humoral theories of disease causation. In 1902, the Montana State Board of Health authorized Louis B. Wilson and Wilson M. Chowning, young pathologists from the University of Minnesota, to investigate spotted fever. Wilson and Chowning conducted an extensive epidemiological study, and their results clearly showed the limitation of cases of the disease to the west side of the valley. Their research also indicated that ticks and their small rodent hosts might be involved in the disease, and because of the high incidence of cases on the west side of the river, it seemed important that these creatures rarely crossed bodies of water such as the Bitterroot River. Although this reasoning was later proved incorrect, it was consistent with contemporary assumptions that dominated the understanding of the germ theory.[15]

Concepts relating to insects or other arthropods as vectors of disease played perhaps the most important role in the early concepts of spotted fever. Zoologists, entomologists, veterinarians, and public health physicians were all interested in tick-borne diseases, and most subscribed to an early model of the process that was later proved wrong. This model postulated that bacteria, which were considered microscopic plants, were transmitted mechanically. For example, the typhoid bacterium was known to be carried on the feet of houseflies from contaminated articles belonging to typhoid patients to the food of potential new hosts. Protozoan organisms—considered to be microscopic animals— were believed to be transmitted biologically by insect and tick bites. Malaria provided the classic case of biological transmission: the organism spent a part of its life cycle developing in the midgut of a mosquito and was transmitted to its human host through a mosquito bite.[16]

The rigid interpretation of this corollary of the germ theory steered spotted fever research at first toward and then away from the conclusion that the disease was tick-borne. Wilson and Chowning announced that they had identified a protozoan organism, which they called *Piroplasma hominis,* in the blood of spotted fever victims. The tick bites reported by patients were thus judged significant because they completed the intellectual construct that related protozoan organisms to biting arthropods.[17] In 1903, however, Charles Wardell Stiles of the Hygienic Laboratory of the U.S. Public Health and Marine Hospital Service reviewed Wilson and Chowning's research but could not find any *Piroplasma.* Being bound himself by the power of the insect vector corollary, Stiles announced that the disease must not be tick-borne because no protozoan organism was involved. He never even considered testing the tick-transmission theory as an independent experiment.[18]

This line of thinking was challenged by University of Chicago investigator Howard Taylor Ricketts, who conducted an experiment to demonstrate that spotted fever was indeed transmissible by ticks.[19] Having shown this, however, Ricketts faced an uphill battle to win acceptance for an etiological organism that was not protozoan in character, a task made more difficult by the characteristics of rickettsiae. Even as late as 1910, after Ricketts had died in Mexico from epidemic typhus (another rickettsial disease that he was studying), a popular book entitled *Insects and Disease* noted that spotted fever was "quite generally believed" to be carried by some sort of protozoan organism.[20]

A second premature conclusion about the germ theory also hampered rapid progress on spotted fever. This was the assumption that all microorganisms shared similar growth and reproduction mechanisms, which rendered all amenable to study with the same techniques. Specifically, the procedure detailed by

Robert Koch in 1884 to demonstrate the tubercle bacillus as the cause of tuberculosis rapidly became accepted as immutable law by a considerable segment of the research community.[21] Commonly called Koch's postulates, these five criteria emphasize the ability to isolate a pure culture of the tubercle bacillus and then to reproduce the disease in an experimental animal after inoculating it with the culture.

Demonstrating that a pure culture was sufficient to produce the disease was only one part of Koch's reasoning about causation, however, and not the most important. For technical reasons, Koch had not been able to use such arguments in his earlier work on anthrax and wound infection or in his concurrent work on cholera.[22] Instead, he had relied on the necessity argument: that if the organism is not present, there is no disease. This argument became the sine qua non of etiological proof because it offered a means for active intervention in the disease process. If the transmission of an organism could be interrupted, no disease would occur.

Many members of the scientific community, however, came to accept a formulation of etiological proof that required cultivation of organisms and demonstration of their ability to cause disease in experimental animals. This rigid adherence to one version of Koch's postulates frustrated many early investigators of spotted fever. Howard Ricketts, who was able to maintain spotted fever in guinea pigs and who believed that he had identified the causative organism under the microscope, tried in vain to cultivate the microbe on lifeless media. He was acutely aware that most of his scientific peers believed culture on lifeless media to be an absolute requirement for proving causation in infectious diseases. His first publication about the putative spotted fever microbe was thus conservatively titled "A Micro-organism Which Apparently Has a Specific Relationship to Rocky Mountain Spotted Fever," and he reminded the secretary of the Montana Board of Health: "We have not been able to cultivate [the microbe], and thus meet one of Koch's great laws. This makes it necessary to bring all kinds of indirect evidence to bear showing that we have the real thing."[23] As with the with the tick-transmission research, Ricketts did not live to see his work vindicated. It was not until 1919, when Simeon Burt Wolbach of Harvard University Medical School published a definitive study of spotted fever, that rickettsiae became widely accepted as causative agents. Even then they remained suspect in some scientific quarters until the late 1930s, when biochemical methods and electron microscopes were introduced.[24]

Although members of the scientific community trained in different specialties constructed spotted fever similarly as a disease caused by a microorganism and transmitted by ticks, internecine rivalries erupted between physicians and entomologists, the two professional groups whose expertise was directly relevant to controlling the new disease. Physicians had controlled other arthropod-borne diseases, such as yellow fever and bubonic plague, and felt that they could handle a tick-borne malady as well. Further, they could treat the victims of the disease and study its bacteriological and pathological aspects. Entomologists had experience eradicating Texas cattle fever, another tick-borne disease, and were experts in the study and control of ticks and insects. They felt confident that they could eliminate the spotted fever tick, and thereby the disease, from the Bitterroot Valley.[25]

In 1902, pathologists Wilson and Chowning sent specimens to Charles Wardell Stiles in Washington, D.C., for his expert determination.[26] In 1904, Stiles named the tick *Dermacentor andersoni* (Stiles) after his colleague John Anderson, the first federal government scientist to publish a study of spotted fever.[27] In June 1908, however, Nathan Banks, a specialist on ticks with the U.S. Bureau of Entomology, published a Department of Agriculture bulletin in which he described and named the Rocky Mountain wood tick *Dermacentor venustus* (Banks).[28] The war of names that subsequently erupted in the professional literature was finally settled in 1923 when the International Commission on Zoological Nomenclature voted to adopt *D. andersoni* as the preferred name.[29] During the intervening years, however, entomologists always called the tick *D. venustus,* and physicians from the U.S. Public Health and Marine Hospital Service always referred to *D. andersoni*. Reports from the two groups appeared side by side in official publications, utilizing the two different names without explanation or apology to readers, who must have been somewhat confused if not already familiar with the controversy.[30]

In sum, the disputes within the scientific community in the early twentieth century were embedded in the larger international intellectual framework shared by all the scientists who investigated Rocky Mountain spotted fever. Since that time, sections of that paradigm have been elaborated as new technologies and concepts have opened fruitful new avenues for research. The fundamental intellectual vision, however, has not changed and continues to determine how scientists construct and interpret new infectious diseases. An examination of the scientific construction of AIDS should illustrate this.

Acquired Immunodeficiency Syndrome (AIDS)

Acquired immunodeficiency syndrome, known primarily by its acronym, AIDS, is an apparently new disease whose name was negotiated by public health leaders to reflect medical understanding of the underlying cause of the varied group of symptoms manifested by patients.[31] It was first recognized by physicians in the United States about 1979 and 1980; the first paper published on the disease appeared in 1981. AIDS has been constructed scientifically as follows: it is caused by a retrovirus, a class of viruses that contain ribonucleic acid, or RNA, as genetic material. A retrovirus utilizes an enzyme known as reverse transcriptase to produce deoxyribonucleic acid, or DNA, within a host cell. This DNA is then incorporated into the DNA that comprises the genome of the host. Once this is accomplished, the retrovirus can reproduce continually as a part of the host's cellular protein synthesis. The AIDS retrovirus, now called HIV for "human immunodeficiency virus," is transmitted from an infected human to a noninfected one through various means that bring infected bodily fluids into contact with the bloodstream of the new host. Examples of such contact include sexual interaction, the birth process, injection of drugs with contaminated needles, transfusion of contaminated blood or blood products, and accidents involving infected blood. Compared with other viral infections, HIV is very difficult to transmit.[32]

AIDS patients often experience a brief period of flulike illness on initial exposure to the virus, after which they may appear healthy for a decade or more. Then, relentlessly, cancers, opportunistic infections, or both appear, often causing wasting and eventually death. As in Rocky Mountain spotted fever, these physiological manifestations are explained within the constructs of the germ theory of infectious diseases and its corollary regarding host immune defenses. For example, a 1993 study of the lymphatic system during the so-called latent period of AIDS revealed that although the victim appears healthy during this time, HIV is debilitating the body's system for fine-screening viruses in the lymph nodes, and it may set into motion a cascade of molecular events that undermine and destroy the immune system. By the time HIV is easily detectable in peripheral blood, immunity has been sufficiently impaired that the patient is unable to resist the microbial invasions and other consequences of immunological breakdown that lead to death.[33]

Like Rocky Mountain spotted fever, AIDS was also characterized initially by its geographical specificity. The earliest cases were reported from the male homosexual, or "gay," communities of Los Angeles, San Francisco, and New York. During 1981 and 1982, the disease was often known as "gay cancer" or "gay-related immune disorder," usually expressed by its acronym, GRID. These names located the disease within the "gay community," an intellectual concept but one that often exhibited geographic specificity within cities.[34] By mid-1982, epidemiological evidence had also linked AIDS to hemophiliacs, intravenous (IV) drug abusers and their sexual partners, and blood transfusion recipients.[35] Although male homosexuals continued to exhibit the highest incidence of AIDS, the names gay cancer and GRID no longer seemed appropriate. Letters and documents generated at the National Institutes of Health (NIH) referred to the disease in early 1982 by the laborious name "Kaposi's sarcoma/opportunistic infections/acquired immunodeficiency syndrome"; by July the name was shortened to "acquired immunodeficiency syndrome" or "acquired immune deficiency syndrome," often with "(Kaposi's sarcoma/opportunistic infections)" added for extra measure.[36] This progression of names reflected the growing conviction within the scientific community that the cancer and the opportunistic infections were symptomatic manifestations of one underlying immune deficiency that apparently was acquired—as opposed to inherited—probably via an infectious agent. The name of the disease thus embodied intellectual perceptions shared by those charged with investigating the disease. These people—often international, national, and local health officials and investigators in university medical schools—held positions of prominence within the scientific medicine establishment.

During the early 1980s, AIDS cases were so rare that standard epidemiological indexes (cases per 100,000 population) provided little useful information in terms of the national picture. Three medical geographers studying AIDS thus developed a figure called the "AIDS quotient," which compared the percentage of any state population with AIDS with the percentage of the entire U.S. population infected with AIDS.[37] Their earliest projection, based on 1984 data from the Centers for Disease Control and Prevention, revealed the heaviest concentrations of AIDS in New York, followed by other northeastern states, Florida, and California.[38] Colorado and Texas were the other western states with significant numbers of cases. Idaho, Montana, Wyoming, Arizona, North and South Dakota, Nebraska, and Iowa were initially untouched by the epidemic. Later data for 1985–88 showed that AIDS had diffused into additional geographical areas.[39] This information does not tell the entire story, of course, because the disease was not distributed evenly within states. It was primarily located in cities with significant high-risk populations.[40] Indeed, a 1993 report by a panel monitoring the social impact of AIDS for the National Research Council declared that "instead of spreading out to the broad American population, as was once feared, HIV is concentrating in pools of persons characterized by poverty, poor health and lack of health care, inadequate education, joblessness, hopelessness, and social disintegration."[41]

The geographical limitation of AIDS to specific social groups was determined largely by behaviors that facilitated transmission of the virus. At first, sexual activities practiced by members of the affected gay communities, especially anal intercourse, provided the most visible route of infection. AIDS-infected hemophiliacs and blood transfusion recipients were often described as "innocent" victims to contrast them with the socially marginalized members of the gay population. Knowledge about AIDS increased, and the incidence of new infections in these two groups dropped dramatically as the former practiced safe sex and the development of an "AIDS test" provided a screening mechanism to protect the blood supply for the latter. A third group of AIDS victims now became the endemic focus for the disease: intravenous drug abusers and their babies, and very poor people, often members of minority groups, living in inner cities. Most of these people lacked political power to force society to pay attention to their problems and were often oblivious to community education efforts. The scientific construction of the disease and associated knowledge about transmission of its causative organism thus were not universally useful in lowering the incidence of AIDS, because the geography of AIDS was most intimately bound up in the *social* construction of the disease, which assigned varying values to the affected groups.

Members of the biomedical research community who sought to comprehend and describe AIDS may have held any of several views about the social meaning of this new disease, but virtually all subscribed to the germ theory of infectious diseases and its corollary about immunity as the intellectual framework within which this new disease was constructed. Abnormal numbers of helper and suppressor T cells provided the first evidence that the underlying pathology of the syndrome was an immune system dysfunction. The "opportunistic" infections and cancers observed in patients previously had been seen almost exclusively in patients whose immune systems had been depleted by disease or suppressed during medical procedures such as organ transplants.[42] As epidemiological evidence accumulated that this immune defect was probably caused by a transmissible agent, investigators adopted a strategy of ruling out known agents.[43] After known pathogens had been eliminated, research on AIDS etiology was guided by the assumption that the unknown agent would be something that attacked T cells. The only such agent known was a newly discovered class of human retroviruses, HTLV-I and HTLV-II, identified in 1980 by Robert C. Gallo and his colleagues at the National Cancer Institute of the U.S. National Institutes of Health.[44] But these retroviruses caused uncontrolled growth in the T cells, producing T cell leukemia. Although the pathogenic process was reversed in AIDS, in that T cells were dying instead of proliferating, the investigators worldwide who began to search for the AIDS agent were primarily retrovirologists looking for a retrovirus because the intellectual paradigm in which they had been schooled predicted that such an organism would be the cause. What Gallo and his associates in Bethesda, Maryland, and Luc Montagnier and his colleagues at the Institut Pasteur in Paris discovered was the retrovirus now called human immunodeficiency virus, or HIV.[45]

Demonstrating the causality of the retrovirus in AIDS, like demonstrating the causality of rickettsiae in Rocky Mountain spotted fever, required the scientific community's consensus on the evidence offered. It is remarkable that the power of the rigid model of Koch's postulates had not abated between the time that Ricketts studied rickettsiae and Montagnier, Gallo, and others studied HIV.[46] The scientific community's objection to HIV as the cause of AIDS rested largely on the supposed failure of HIV to meet Koch's postulates. Molecular biologist Peter Duesberg and physiologist Robert Root-Bernstein each wrote critiques of HIV as the cause of AIDS based on the presumed failure of the virus to meet Koch's postulates.[47] But each man defined Koch's postulates in their most rigid form and ignored their role as techniques to satisfy the requirements of scientific logic. Each emphasized AIDS researchers' inability to demonstrate HIV in every case of AIDS, the fact that every sexual partner of HIV-infected people did not also develop AIDS, and other examples of exceptions to the logical position that HIV is sufficient to cause the disease. In contrast, the scientists who argued for HIV as the cause of AIDS invoked the necessity argument: in the absence of HIV, AIDS does not occur.[48]

A taxonomic tempest much like the one described in relation to Rocky Mountain spotted fever erupted over the name of the AIDS retrovirus. Montagnier's group at the Institut Pasteur isolated a retrovirus from tissue obtained from an AIDS patient with swollen lymph nodes; hence they called their putative AIDS organism "lymphadenophy-associated virus," or LAV.[49] In Bethesda, Gallo's group initially perceived their retrovirus as related to the two other human T cell lymphotrophic retroviruses they had identified; hence they called it "human-T-cell lymphotrophic virus III," or HTLV-III.[50] By 1985 these two agents had been shown to be identical.[51] A priority dispute erupted, however, along with a dispute over patent rights to the diagnostic test produced in each laboratory. A Nobel Prize might be at stake, and there was never any question that millions of dollars would be made from the AIDS test. Publications from each laboratory therefore called the virus by the name each had given it. Out of respect for the unresolved conflict, and wanting to communicate clearly, other AIDS scientists began using both names in their publications. The editorial policies of major journals revealed both nationalistic feelings and the personal views of editors. Journals published in France and others that supported the French claim always referred to the virus as LAV/HTLV-III; those that supported the U.S. claim used HTLV-III/LAV. Those not embroiled in the controversy found the entire matter unduly laborious. In May 1986, a multinational committee suggested in letters to the editors of *Science* and *Nature* that the name "human immunodeficiency virus" was both more descriptive and less cumbersome than the other two versions.[52] The fact that two prestigious scientific journals of record were used to announce the name change underscores the commonality of intellectual constructs regarding AIDS across international boundaries. Both the Gallo and Montagnier laboratories agreed with the proposal, and the new name was adopted.

Scientific Construction of New Diseases

Having examined the geographical and intellectual "places" where Rocky Mountain spotted fever and AIDS were first defined, what can we say about how scientists view new diseases? First, geographical place is most important when the disease is initially identified. Both lay and medical observers may tie disease symptoms—in this case, spotted fever and immune deficiency—to the place where they were first observed: the Rocky Mountain region and the gay communities of large cities. Names that link diseases to the first reported location may or may not endure. Additional information may prove that geography is indeed important in determining disease incidence (as in spotted fever), but if the link is not clear or if it is socially defined (as in AIDS), geography will figure more prominently in the social construction of the disease and may become a negligible factor in the scientific construction.

Following the initial period of disease identification, scientific concepts about pathogenesis and etiology emerge within the intellectual framework of the germ theory and its corollaries. The individual experiences of investigators may generate differences of opinion. Furthermore, scientists may uncritically accept the apparent implications of particular facets of the theory even when those implications are buttressed by little evidence. Investigators usually find an etiological agent that satisfies the requirements according to their understanding of the germ theory. The putative agent may or may not prove valid after further research. The most creative and successful investigators are those who can see beyond the limitations of the paradigm, who understand that it provides a framework for investigation rather than a set of rules to which research results must conform.

Perhaps most revealing of the power of this intellectual model are the disputes that emerge because of internecine rivalry. Differences among scientists on this level may lead to priority disputes as well as annoying and, in retrospect, almost comical pettiness. These disputes are based, however, on a shared belief about biological reality. Only the details of who got there first are in question. Such rivalry may impede the elaboration of scientific knowledge about a disease, but it rarely stops it.

In sum, the germ theory of infectious diseases and its corollaries have framed the scientific construction of infectious diseases in the twentieth century. The transformation from the older humoral view to the contemporary paradigm is so complete, in fact, that the assumptions inherent in the germ theory are essentially accepted as scientific facts, both by historians and by medical researchers. Nonscientists may not comprehend the differences between rickettsiae and retroviruses, but the concept that microscopic and submicroscopic organisms cause disease goes virtually unchallenged. In the scientific construction of Rocky Mountain spotted fever, the disease is not caused by Rocky Mountain air, water, or other aspects of place. It results from the conjunction of the causative organism with susceptible human hosts via the bite of an infected tick living within that suitable habitat. Similarly, AIDS results not from living in particular geographic locales but from behaviors that promote viral transmission among infected people who may be concentrated in those locales. The connection of disease with place—in the mountain West as elsewhere—has in the twentieth century been transformed from a causative bond to a situational association.

6 "Many Have Died and Others Must"

The Silicosis Epidemic in Western Hardrock

Mining, 1900–1925

ALAN DERICKSON

Silicosis, a chronic respiratory disorder caused by the inhalation of dust containing free silica, was widespread among the workforce of the metal-mining industry in the mountain West in the early twentieth century. Salient aspects of the silicosis problem illuminate distinctive characteristics of this region. Indeed, diverse economic, social, political, and environmental factors present in the industrializing mountain West plainly had a strong, even decisive, influence on the health status of the hardrock miners who constituted a significant share of the population of several states, including Nevada, throughout this period.

By focusing on the exceptional nature of regional development in this case, we also clarify miners' silicosis as an epidemiological phenomenon during rapid industrialization. In this particular set of circumstances, it is curiously appropriate to describe the occurrence of the disease as an epidemic. At a glance, it might seem more fitting to consider as endemic, not epidemic, a common chronic condition limited to a region, and within this region largely confined to certain localities. Shouldn't the term *epidemic* be reserved for dramatic outbreaks of infectious diseases such as cholera and bubonic plague?

Charles Rosenberg's cogent brief for a narrow construction of the concept of epidemic notwithstanding, there are good reasons to call metal miners' pneumoconiosis in the period 1900–25 an epidemic. A broad conceptualization of what constitutes an epidemic certainly enjoys considerable support in the field of public health. In its manual for health officers, the American Public Health Association (APHA) defines an epidemic as "the occurrence in a community or region of cases of an illness (or an outbreak) clearly in excess of expectancy." As Judith Mausner and Anita Bahn have pointed out, this definition is expansive in two ways. First, it sets no numerical threshold for the number of cases required to constitute an epidemic. Instead, the APHA defines the phenomenon in terms of a departure from expectations, expectations that necessarily are formed from past experience with the disease. That is to say that history enters directly into epidemiological reasoning at this juncture, as at so many others in the biomedical sciences. Second, under the APHA definition, an epidemic may, as Mausner and Bahn note, "encompass any time period." Similarly, in their textbook *Epidemiology: Principles and Methods,* Brian MacMahon and Thomas F. Pugh explain that an epidemic need not occur "within a period as short as a few days or weeks."[1] Considered in the light of this broad interpretation, the dread disease of western mining looks even more dreadful.

Sometime in the second half of the nineteenth century, in the wake of the rise of large-scale extractive activity, silicosis emerged as an occupational disease with significant frequency. In the absence of vital statistics from the mountain states, it is impossible to gauge the magnitude of the problem with precision. Nonetheless, the extant anecdotal reports certainly are suggestive. In 1893, journalist Dan De Quille, an acute observer of the Comstock silver mines and their workers, made this unhappy assessment: "Death stalks through the dark chambers of the mines in a thousand shapes. Generally his blows are sudden and terrible. More pitiable, however, seems the living death of the doomed man lingering down to the tomb in the never-relaxed clutch of miners' consumption." Given the relatively primitive technology deployed in the initial stages of mining development, and given what we know about the relatively small doses of dust generated by this technology, it seems reasonable to assume that a fairly small number of cases of pneumoconiosis manifested themselves in the western mining centers during this time.[2] Before the turn of the century, this pattern of scattered cases confined to mining localities and occurring at what appears to have been a more or less constant rate made miners' silicosis an endemic disorder.

    After the turn of the century, however, morbidity and mortality from silicosis soared above this baseline, exceeding greatly the expected rates of illness. The primary cause of this accelerating rate of disease was technological. In the closing decades of the nineteenth century, the methods of ore extraction and processing advanced considerably. Of greatest importance were the substitution of dynamite for black powder as an explosive and the dissemination of power drills rather than hand drills for boring the holes into which explosive charges were placed. As of 1902, drills driven by electricity or steam were deployed in more than 70 percent of gold and silver ore mining and in more than 80 percent of copper ore mining. After the latency period between dust exposure and the manifestation of symptoms of illness had passed, an epidemic of industrial disease broke out across the broad region between the Rockies and the Sierra Nevada. Indeed, many contemporary observers immediately attributed the rise in occupational lung disease to technological innovation. An editorial in *Engineering and Mining Journal,* a leading trade publication, in 1904 noted that "miner's consumption has only assumed prominence since the introduction of power drills, which produce a far greater amount of dust than when the work is done by hand. Moreover," added the editorialist, reflecting on the uneven, breakthrough-and-bottleneck character of innovation, "in the hurry to push forward exploitation, insufficient time is given for the dust to settle after blasting." Techniques for treating ore following its extraction also became more mechanized in the late nineteenth century. The new techniques threw much more dust into the working environment and pulverized rock into smaller particles capable of penetrating to the furthest depths of the lungs, where microscopic bits of silicious rock cause the greatest damage.[3] Industrialization thus converted an endemic condition into an epidemic.

According to the APHA definition of an epidemic, the commencement of the silicosis epidemic should be marked by a significant upturn in incidence as reported in vital statistics or some other source of quantitative data. Unfortunately, no body of valid data allowing a comparison of the incidence of silicosis in the late nineteenth century with incidence in the early twentieth century exists.[4] Fortunately, however, it is possible to periodize this problem the old-fashioned way, by noting the occurrence of the kind of dramatic outbreak that is usually associated with infectious conditions.

The initial outbreak, an extremely virulent one, took place in eastern Nevada. In a remote canyon in Lincoln County, ranchers stumbled on rich deposits of gold in 1890. After a sample of ore assayed at $1,000 per ton, a small rush of prospectors descended on the site. Within a few years, Joseph R. DeLaMar, a colorful Dutch entrepreneur, had taken control of this small boom by purchasing mining claims and building an ore-processing mill. DeLaMar, a former ship captain, immigrated to the United States in the 1860s and first became involved in precious metals extraction in Leadville, Colorado, in the 1870s. An experienced, highly astute mining investor, he understood the need to process ore right at the mine. The mine's isolated desert location, a hundred miles from the nearest rail line, made hauling out wagon loads of rock prohibitively expensive. Hence, DeLaMar had a sizable, modern mill in operation by early 1895. By the end of June 1895, the DeLaMar Nevada Gold Mining Company was shipping $30,000 worth of concentrated gold and silver ore per week.[5]

The budding mining town, which soon took the name Delamar, lacked both a connection to the railroad network and a local supply of water. (The closest water was sixteen miles away.) Unable to wet down the rock as it was being milled, DeLaMar chose to crush and grind it into a fine powder in a completely dry state. This turned out to be a disastrous decision for the mill workers. The quartzite rock that held the gold was highly silicious. Indeed, the formation in this district was approximately 80 percent free silica. As ore extraction increased, milling operations naturally grew apace. Soon DeLaMar's mill was treating three hundred tons of ore per day.[6]

The sixty or so workers inside the processing plant breathed air thoroughly contaminated with microscopic, respirable silica particles. Needless to say, there are no quantitative data on the dust concentrations in the plant, but nontechnical reports give a rough sense of the magnitude of the hazard. "The air is filled with an impalpable dust and in portions of the mill it is so dense that one can not be recognized a few feet away," noted one observer. Another recalled that "an electric light ten feet away looked like a fire bug, the air was so full of dust." The dusty room through which masses of powdered quartzite passed on an unenclosed conveyor belt became known as "the death trap."[7]

The intense respiratory hazard was catastrophic to the health of the mill workers. In this instance the impact of industrialization was so strong that the disease entity itself transmuted into an acute form. To make clear the extraordinary difference between the two forms of the disease, consider the typical trajectory of chronic silicosis. A cumulative-dose disorder, this type of pneumoconiosis generally manifests itself only after ten or more years of regular inhalation of mineral dust. Often miners worked twenty or thirty years in the presence of this insidious hazard before experiencing shortness of breath, cough, and chest pain. Following the onset of these symptoms, respiratory capacity would slowly deteriorate over the course of many years, usually as the partially disabled miner continued to work. Thus, silicosis has generally been considered a chronic disorder of aging workers, incurred after decades of working in a dusty environment.[8]

The gradual descent characteristic of chronic silicosis contrasts sharply with the precipitous fall of the employees of the Delamar mill. The pioneering investigation mounted at the end of the 1890s by William W. Betts provides a remarkable profile of acute silicosis in this group. Apparently acting at his own initiative, motivated by scientific curiosity and humanitarian concern, Betts, a Salt Lake City physician, explored the ore workers' plight using the traditional methods of "shoe-leather epidemiology." From data gathered on thirty fatal cases, he determined that the average pneumoconiosis victim died twenty-nine months after first entering the Delamar mill. In ten cases, the duration of actual dust exposure was nine months or less. The average victim died at thirty years of age; one individual in the sample succumbed at the age of twenty. Betts estimated that through 1899, "conservatively speaking, about a hundred have already died . . . [including] six that I know of in the past two months." Less cautiously, David Farmer, an activist for the Western Federation of Miners, contended in a Labor Day speech in 1899 that the Delamar mill had caused more fatalities to Americans than had the war in the Philippines. At about the same time, in a surprising departure from the "speak no evil" booster customs of mining-town journalism, the Delamar newspaper reported as an undisputed fact that rock dust had killed at least three hundred mill employees.[9]

Unquestionably, Betts's report, published in January 1900 in the eminent and widely read *Journal of the American Medical Association,* did much to force broader recognition of the growing silicosis epidemic. Yet this revelation depended on extraordinary exertions by Dr. Betts, who assiduously collected data on silicotics dispersed over a wide area. Although the typical victim survived only eight months after leaving his job in Delamar, this interval afforded ample time for dying men to scatter in all directions in search of family support and other assistance to deal with the incurable progressive disorder. "A great many of the men were from adjoining states and the far East," Betts observed. "Many would return to their distant homes as soon as they were broken in health, and it is difficult to keep track of them, though many have died and others must." The Salt Lake physician found that "almost every town in Nevada and southern Utah has had its victim," including eleven deaths within a year in St. George, Utah, alone. Where no one stepped forward to undertake more of this sort of aggressive case finding, silicosis, at least as an epidemic, went unrecognized or underrecognized. Indeed, the desperate flight of disabled mine and mill workers from hardrock mining districts served to obscure the true magnitude of the dust-generated disease epidemic that occurred during this period.[10]

In the aftermath of the Delamar disaster, evidence mounted for the adverse consequences of inhaling rock dust. Over the course of the ensuing decade, both lay and professional observations of diverse facets of the epidemic accumulated. In general the 1900s witnessed an awareness of the predisposition of advanced silicosis cases to develop tuberculosis, although the Delamar mill employees succumbed before they had a chance to contract this infection as a complication. At the same time, however, clinicians and other close observers in the hardrock mining communities began to differentiate tuberculosis, or consumption, from a "miners' consumption" that was not contagious and did not produce night sweats and some of the other major symptoms of tuberculosis. Unfortunately, despite the dissemination of this crucial analytical distinction, the prevailing terminology, used by physicians and nonphysicians alike, continued to perpetuate confusion through the early 1920s. The name "miners' consumption" was loosely applied both to silicosis, the simple form of pneumoconiosis, and to silico-tuberculosis, the complicated form of the disorder.[11]

The proliferation of medical case reports and informal accounts of illness brought pressure for more extensive inquiry into miners' respiratory disorders. So did provocative, if casual, estimates of the magnitude of the epidemic. For example, in 1911 two longtime Montana copper workers told a state legislative committee that approximately one-third of the men who had spent their whole careers in the Butte mines suffered from miners' consumption. Demands for research intensified in the wake of epidemiological findings of widespread pneumoconiosis in metal-mining districts in South Africa, Britain, and Australia during the first decade of the century. Seemingly, Betts's one-man initiative plus the accumulated anecdotal reports had set the stage for a full-scale epidemiological study.[12]

Yet no investigation was immediately forthcoming. Instead, the dynamics of chronic-disease recognition were shaped by political and economic factors peculiar to this mining region. The state health apparatus in the mountain West was very weak, and employees of state health departments had only minimal expertise. In contrast to states like Massachusetts and New York, which had abundant medical resources, the western mining states were unprepared to pursue the matter. Rather than the reformist, even crusading, scientism so common to the Progressive Era, raw class politics drove the process of knowledge generation in this setting. With their long-standing fears about lung disease substantiated by episodes like the Delamar disaster, hardrock workers began to agitate for government regulation of dust exposure, even in the absence of conclusive quantitative studies.

This movement for corrective legislation was led by that notorious band of radical unionists, the Western Federation of Miners (WFM). In the two decades after the union's founding in Butte, Montana, in 1893, numerous encounters involving dynamite and various forms of artillery established the WFM as the most militant labor organization in North America.[13] Though hardly a learned society dedicated to the production of scientific knowledge, the WFM nonetheless contributed significantly to the process of disease recognition. By its strenuous insistence on ameliorative measures, the union further raised the visibility of the issue of work-induced dust disease and thus added to the pressure for epidemiological research.

Initially, the union called for underground ventilation standards. In 1908, John Lowney, a WFM activist in Montana, argued that only government intervention could create a healthful working environment. Lowney drew on his personal knowledge of conditions in the Butte copper mines to put the matter forward in vivid terms:

We have humane societies for the protection of animals with agents paid by the state, but there is no society, humane or otherwise, which deems it worth while to inquire into the conditions under which human beings work in the mines of Butte. They take no notice of the daily processions on the streets of Butte, wending their way to the cemeteries, and those who are borne in those processions to their last resting place have been the very flower of physical manhood stricken in their prime by that dread disease known as miners' consumption. . . .

Those conditions can be changed to a great extent by proper ventilation and better sanitary methods, but those things cost money[,] and human life, here as elsewhere, is the cheapest thing in all the world. We need legislation to enforce better sanitary conditions in our mines.

Three years later, the Montana legislature responded to the union pressure by passing a mine ventilation statute. A number of loopholes rendered the law useless, however. The most vitiating flaw was the absence of a precise quantitative standard for underground air flow.[14]

After the bitter experience of this illusory reform, the union shifted its objective. Beginning in 1912, it primarily advocated legislation for wet methods of dust abatement. By the 1910s, power drilling equipment that featured hollow drills through which water was injected to suppress dust at its source was widely available. Accordingly, in the inaugural session of the Arizona state legislature in 1912, the WFM pushed through a protective measure providing that "where necessary an adequate spraying system shall be installed and used to settle dust." But this statute, too, contained a debilitating loophole: it failed to specify the circumstances under which such dust abatement was mandatory. The following year, Arizona lawmakers responded to further lobbying from the miners' organization by repairing this deficiency. The amended mining law obliged mine operators to use water whenever they extracted dry ore with mechanical drills.[15] During the industrializing era in the United States, this sort of political intervention to dictate a change in the actual methods of production (and not merely to require a guardrail or enclosure around a dangerous operation) was quite extraordinary.[16]

The union launched a similarly audacious drive for reform in Nevada. In mid-1912, WFM Local 121 in Tonopah wrote a bill that mandated not just wet drilling but also wet handling of ore during shoveling and other dust-raising activities. Before the next legislative session, both the Nevada Board of Health and the state inspector of mines publicly endorsed the proposal. The mine inspector, Edward Ryan, made a particularly emphatic appeal for reform. Ryan began by asserting that his own observations and reports from other knowledgeable observers in the mining camps confirmed that miners' consumption constituted a "great menace to the lives of those working in mines and ore houses," and then argued for the enactment of the dust control plan initiated by the

Tonopah Miners' Union. "This is a question of vital importance," Ryan concluded, "and I cannot too strongly urge the members of the next Legislature to give it careful study, to the end that something may be done to stop this withering blight."[17] The combination of such authoritative support with the considerable political clout of the miners' union led the Nevada legislature to enact protective measures for both drilling and ore handling in the 1913 session.[18]

In addition to its efforts toward primary prevention of silicosis, the WFM also opened a second front in the battle against occupational disease. Commencing in 1914, the organization demanded that workers' compensation programs provide benefits for this work-induced disorder, just as they did for traumatic injuries incurred on the job. In broaching this issue, union president Charles Moyer provocatively referred to "the prevalence of miners' consumption, caused by dust-laden air in all mines." Tellingly, Moyer assumed a widespread prevalence of the disease and considered such a prevalence necessary to justify the legislation, but he did not venture any firm estimate of the number of disabled men entitled to claim compensation.[19]

After the enactment of regulatory measures in Nevada and Arizona and the initiation of the campaign for workers' compensation coverage, federal health officials somewhat belatedly took up the challenge of determining the magnitude of the silicosis problem in the hardrock mining industry. Although rigorous and systematic by the standards of the time, the federal epidemiological studies were limited in several ways. All suffered from self-selection bias. All were confounded by the flight of a substantial proportion of the advanced silicotics from mining districts. All were merely descriptive in nature, making no real attempt to estimate a dose-response relationship.[20]

Somewhat curiously, the preliminary reconnaissance in the Rocky Mountain West proved to be abortive. In 1911 the U.S. Public Health and Marine Hospital Service (which became the U.S. Public Health Service the following year) sent a member of its medical staff, Samuel Hotchkiss, to investigate working conditions in Colorado. Although Hotchkiss apparently performed no medical examinations himself, he did review death certificates and other local records. By this exercise, he found evidence to suggest that miners' consumption prevailed widely in Colorado's metal-mining communities.[21]

Rather than pursue the problem in Colorado, a center of militant unionism, federal officials chose to launch their first major epidemiological investigation in Joplin, Missouri, apparently a safe haven of nonunion tranquillity. During 1915, the Public Health Service (PHS) screened 720 lead-zinc workers in southwestern Missouri and found that 60 percent had miners' consumption. After allowing for self-selection and other sources of bias, Dr. Anthony J. Lanza, the principal investigator in this study, estimated that at least 30 percent of the area's miners had silicosis or silico-tuberculosis, a shocking finding.[22]

The second major federal investigation of this phenomenon took place between 1916 and 1919 in Butte, Montana, at that time one of the world's great mining centers. Approximately fifteen thousand workers were employed in copper ore extraction during the World War I boom. Daniel Harrington, a mining engineer with the U.S. Bureau of Mines (BOM), took dozens of measurements of the dust hazard in the area. As in Joplin, the silica concentration in the labyrinthine workings beneath Butte commonly reached extremely high levels. For example, in the Mountain View mine of the Anaconda Copper Mining Company, Harrington drew sixty-six air samples in diverse work situations. He found that rock dust averaged more than 60 percent free silica and that the average particulate concentration was sixty-five milligrams per cubic meter of air. This level of air contamination exceeds today's federal Mine Safety and Health Administration permissible exposure limit by approximately four hundred times. Commenting on rank-and-file consciousness of this severe health threat, Harrington reported that workers "very generally understood" that working in poorly ventilated sections of the Mountain View mine was "merely a form of slow suicide."[23]

Although the design of the Butte study called for considerable environmental monitoring, this concern did not extend to an attempt to determine the dust exposure of individual miners participating in the study so that individual cumulative dust doses could be calculated. That is to say, the project failed to integrate all the causal factors involved so as to delineate a dose-response relationship. Although it thus remained largely a descriptive and somewhat disjointed exercise, the study did provide powerful evidence of substantial dust inhalation by virtually all types of underground workers. Collecting medical data in facilities provided by the Butte Anti-Tuberculosis Society, Lanza appears to have used essentially the same clinical workup that he used in Joplin—medical and occupational histories, a physical examination, and a chest X-ray. In the fifteen months up through February 1918, he and Dr. Royd Sayers examined 1,018 mine workers. The PHS physicians diagnosed 432, or 42.8 percent, of the miners as silicotic. Due to the usual self-selection bias and a number of other complicating factors, the Public Health Service was unable to determine the true prevalence of silicosis in Butte. Nonetheless, we can assume that, even with a prevalence well below 42 percent, a substantial amount of pneumoconiosis existed in this mining district.[24]

Taken together, the Joplin and Butte investigations succeeded in clarifying the causes of silicosis and its extent across the metal-mining workforce. Given these gains in knowledge, the surgeon general concluded that "future studies should be confined to establishing the presence of the disease in any particular territory."[25] In line with this shift to a more modest objective, the PHS and the BOM undertook less elaborate screening projects in western hardrock communities after the Butte study was completed. In one of these projects, Dr. Cleve E. Kindall ventured to Tonopah, Nevada, in 1921 to examine gold miners. Promotional announcements of the project urged "as many men as possible to come in for chest examinations, not only those who fear that their lungs are affected by the dust, but also those whose lungs are unimpaired." Nonetheless, self-selection by those with clinical manifestations of disease definitely took place in Tonopah, too. Kindall found that fully 80 percent (244 of 303) of the mine workers he studied there had silicosis.[26] In contrast, two similar projects in the early 1920s found much lower percentages. In Oatman, Arizona, a PHS-BOM investigation found that 33 of 112 (29 percent) hardrock workers showed signs of dust disease. Likewise, in the Mother Lode of California, 45 of 181 (25 percent) gold miners were diagnosed with silicosis in 1921–22.[27]

After 1922, the federal government discontinued this series of field studies and turned its attention to other pneumoconioses, such as byssinosis and anthracosis. Although they conducted epidemiological inquiries in numerous western mining centers, the Bureau of Mines and the Public Health Service abandoned the study without making any estimate of the overall prevalence of silicosis in the region. By a very rough estimate, it seems reasonable to believe that about 20 percent of western hardrock workers suffered from the disorder; in other words, there were at least thirty thousand silicotic miners at any given time during the first quarter of this century.[28]

In contrast to its dramatic arrival at the Delamar mill, there appears to have been no decisive endpoint to the pneumoconiosis epidemic. Nonetheless, the problem in the western mines seems to have declined somewhat after 1925. Without uncritically accepting the operators' assurances that the hazard was simply eliminated by the 1920s, we can see signs that hazard prevention measures implemented in the 1910s were having an effect a decade later. Dust control came as a result of wet-methods legislation, improved mechanical ventilation, and, perhaps most important, growing awareness of the simple fact that wet drilling cuts rock faster than dry drilling. Just as technological change had given rise to an elevated rate of pneumoconiosis, further technological change (often in response to statutory requirements) gradually mitigated the dust hazard and reduced the incidence of work-induced respiratory disease. Although a significant silicosis problem persisted, and new cases were generated by the dusty conditions that remained in many mines, it appears that this disorder returned to a state of endemicity in the metal mines of the mountain West after 1925. Because it was largely the product of highly variable technological, economic, and political factors, miners' silicosis (like all other diseases) was not a static epidemiological phenomenon. Moreover, like all other occupational diseases, it was created by humans and therefore could be controlled, even eradicated, by human agency.[29]

7   Frontier Nursing

The Deaconess Experience in Montana, 1890–1960

PIERCE C. MULLEN

We have tried to emphasize that the development of the modern nurse has been closely allied with the rising status of women. Wherever women have had very little freedom, nursing has had difficulty developing as a profession. Modern nursing has depended upon the development of modern medicine and the hospital. We believe that the individual most responsible for the development of modern medicine is the nurse.[1]

And there was the utter void created by the longing—ineradicable, unremitting, pervasive—for the warmth of human contact. A warm smile and an outstretched hand were valued even above the offerings of modern science, but the later were far more accessible than the former.[2]

These two observations bracket the story of nursing in the western tradition. Just as the history of the West is currently being reinterpreted, so is the history of nursing; in both, issues of gender are emerging as crucial. The frontier nursing experience is an important part of the general history of nursing and shares its grand themes: the rigorous duty to preserve health; the recovery of mental and physical soundness insofar as science, practice, and social values permit; and the continuing search for theoretical and clinical means to achieve recovery.

The story of the Deaconess movement in Montana is the story of nursing practices in frontier America in microcosm. Accidents, sickness, and mental disease were common to all frontier settlements, and miners, ranchers, and other residents all felt a human need for nurses. Nursing sisterhoods responded to that need: a number of different Roman Catholic nursing orders were present on the frontier, as were a few Anglican sisterhoods, the Deaconesses of several Protestant mainline churches, and hardy individuals who responded to the vocation and practiced in the West.[3] In sum, the frontier was a missionary frontier as well as an economic and social one.

The need for nurses on the frontier was readily apparent, and numerous nursing sisterhoods responded. When Father de Smet invited the Sisters of Charity of Leavenworth to come to Last Chance Gulch (in Helena, Montana) in 1870, the sisters had already received requests for help from Denver,

Leadville, and other Colorado communities. Several western Ontario nursing schools had become involved in sending women west. And although it is not widely known or discussed, several female physicians from this province had begun to practice in the region as well. Their story is an interesting one: when their transitory communities became better established, male physicians arrived who then frequently married these pioneering women. Often the women doctors then became nurses in their husbands' practices.[4] Each of the nursing sisterhoods left an imprint on Montana. Isolated settlements required on-site facilities to care for those who could not care for themselves, and the list of Montana hospitals and clinics is almost as long as the state's boundaries are distant.[5]

The Deaconess experience is an encapsulation of this larger account. What brought the Deaconesses to the West? In a word, Christian missionary vocations were the engine driving the movement. Methodist clergymen concerned about the health of their flocks issued persistent calls for help. The Deaconesses responded, filled with a missionary zeal to serve the spiritual needs of the sick through medical care. In this service, their own spirituality would, they hoped, also grow.

Their belief and zeal would serve these nurses well, but the secular demands on them were quite complicated, too. Once they arrived they faced every practical difficulty the frontier had to offer: vast distance, unremitting work, and few helpers. Much attention had to be spent on finding and training new recruits for the cause. By the time the territories of the frontier West attained statehood in an industrialized nation, medicine was becoming more science than art and nurses increasingly were required to learn new procedures, skills, and ideas. As if the challenge of facing new theories, therapeutics, and practices was not enough, new forms of organization and licensure were articulated and developed.[6] Obviously, becoming a nurse meant something different to the generations that succeeded this pioneering wave. Nevertheless, as poorly salaried as it was, and as difficult as it was to achieve for many young women, nursing was a move up in status; it was a profession.

Practical and Spiritual Traditions

The twin pillars on which the Methodist Deaconess movement rested were the Nightingale tradition in England and the experiences of Pastor Theodor Fliedner in Kaiserwerth, Germany. The Nightingale school was a strict and hierarchical model of nursing instruction and commitment. The students, called nurse probationers, were expected to work long hours, live and eat in dormitory accommodations, and account for every minute of their day. It incorporated the British class system and craft apprenticeship instructional techniques.

Nurse probationers who could afford to pay for their board, room, and instruction were offered medical lectures by physicians. The less fortunate women received a modest stipend and signed on for a work period of three to five years, which enabled the institution to recoup its expenses and remain self-sustaining. The Methodist Deaconess leadership adopted and modified this model as a realistic means of instructing young women. The nurse director was more than a matron: she was a paradigm of deportment, commitment, and spiritual concern for the individual probationer.[7]

If Britain provided the practical basis for bringing the novice into the mainstream of practice, the Kaiserwerth program became the spiritual basis for Deaconess training. Pastor Fliedner had seen the tremendous concern for the sick and the poor among the Mennonites in Holland and translated what he had witnessed into his own life and work. In his view, the externals of nursing care were secondary to the spiritual light within. Healing was a religious function as well as a housekeeping chore. Each patient had to be made aware of the soul within, of the possibility of salvation on a transcendent level. Nurses required medical training, of course, but they must offer more. They must carry the divine spirit to the suffering.[8]

The practical and spiritual traditions on which Deaconess training was based must have aroused some internal conflicts in those first-generation frontier nurses. An enlightened suffragist herself, and a gifted scholar, Florence Nightingale combined social know-how with a remarkable drive to secure a niche for nurses independent of outside meddling—and that included the British medical establishment. Pastor Fliedner's more quietistic view was almost medieval in its acceptance of inner transformation. The student nurse was to experience a personal manifestation of God's will in the patient through healing and recovery, or in decline and death. Both models, the British and the German, stressed duty, self-sacrifice, and upright and moral deportment. A nurse must be psychologically able to stand independently and present her views in a forthright manner. The result was that until scientific medicine made it impossible to continue without extensive academic training, novices were given a quasi-religious indoctrination rather than a medical one. Echoes of this tradition remained in nursing instruction in Montana's Methodist hospitals, although such views increasingly became historical genuflections. Between 1902 and the mid-1920s, however, nurse trainees lived in a cloistered environment. Their personal recollections of girlish pranks are reminiscent of seminary humor.[9]

In the United States, Protestant nursing sisterhoods, most based on the Nightingale canon, began to emerge just before the Civil War. To avoid anti-Catholic bias (and most of the originators of these Protestant groups admired the work of the Catholic sisters), all were called Deaconesses. The Methodist Deaconesses were a peculiarly American amalgamation of secular philanthropic spirit and traditional practices of the convent. Some chose to marry, others, particularly among the leaders, remained single. All were expected to conform to a certain level of spiritual and ethical behavior.

The Methodist church sent capable missionaries to the frontier West. In 1896, the son of Rev. F. A. Riggin, a Methodist minister in the Great Falls area, became ill. There was no Protestant hospital, and Riggin was evidently dismayed at the thought of sending his son to the new Catholic establishment, Columbus Hospital. In the late summer of that year the Montana Methodist Mission met in Sand Coulee. A committee of three ministers was authorized to establish a hospital in Great Falls: Riggin, Rev. O. W. Mintzer, and Rev. W. W. "Brother Van" van Orsdel, a missionary who would play a critical role in Methodist nursing in the state. The three worked efficiently: Great Northern magnate J. J. Hill donated land, others contributed money, and the hospital opened in 1898 as Deaconess (later Great Falls Deaconess) Hospital. Financial difficulties appeared almost immediately. Initial optimism had led to the appointment of administrators inadequate to the task, but "neither the preachers nor trustees could have produced the desired results." Miss E. Augusta Ariss, "a competent and sacrificial leader," [10] was sent by the Methodist City, Home, and Foreign Missions Office in Chicago to restore an appropriate Protestant presence.

Mrs. Lucy Rider Meyer, the founder of the Deaconess organization, selected a formidable character in E. Augusta Ariss. Miss Ariss, as she was always called, was a graduate of the two-year program at Guelph General Hospital Nurses' Training School. She served for two years as a Deaconess novice in Chicago under Mrs. Meyer, and then served five years at the Fred Victor Rescue Mission in the slums of Toronto, where she became a well-known figure as she peddled around on her three-wheeled cycle. Officially she was loaned by the Chicago headquarters to the Northern Montana Mission for two years; she remained for nearly thirty. [11]

Her regimen in Great Falls became the ideal for all Deaconess hospitals: mandatory daily chapel attendance, participation in prayer meetings at the nurses' quarters on Saturday evening, attendance at morning prayers before going on duty at 7:00 A.M., and daily hymn singing at 7:00 P.M. Miss Ariss reported in her biennial review for 1917–19 that "the object of training schools in general may be said to be the training of nurses for service in their profession; the object of the Montana Deaconess Hospital is the training of Nurses for CHRISTIAN service." [12]

Miss Ariss saw these duties as ancillary to her supervision of the nursing department of the hospital and, in general, to her governance of the total hospital operation. In order to pay off the debt she had inherited, she expanded the facility, often surrendering her own bed to provide additional space for patients.

Her thrift was legendary. She had found ten safety pins when she came. Each patient was obliged to account for any used, and she kept them in a safe until they were required for use once again. In her pedagogical role she paid close attention to the work being pursued at St. Luke's in New York and at Johns Hopkins hospital in Baltimore. In keeping with her Deaconess background, she always built new doctrine on the foundation of the principles of the Nightingale Pledge:

> I solemnly pledge myself before God and in the presence of this assembly:
>   To pass my life in purity and to practice my profession faithfully. I will abstain from whatever is deleterious and mischievous, and will not take or knowingly administer any harmful drug. I will do all in my power to elevate the standard of my profession, and will hold in confidence all personal matters committed to my keeping and all family affairs coming to my knowledge in the practice of my profession. With loyalty will I endeavor to aid the physician in his work, and devote myself to the welfare of those committed to my care.[13]

These tireless efforts combined with the work of active bishops to create seven Deaconess hospitals. Miss Ariss began the Montana training program with a couple of volunteers recruited from the eastern states. For about a decade she struggled to maintain a semblance of intellectual rigor, even providing an occasional lecture at the bedside of a patient.

The gulf between physician and nurse was wide and deep, and nurse trainees were generally thought of as odd but useful servants rather than professional health care providers.[14] To address the professional character of nursing, Miss Ariss worked diligently to build institutional reinforcements for her people. Alumnae were formed into the Montana State Association of Graduate Nurses in 1915, which shortly thereafter became affiliated with the American Nurses' Association. In a state that reveled, and revels still, in hands-on politicking, she organized a nursing headquarters in the state capitol building. She worked with her Catholic colleagues to establish a state board of examiners in 1913, and not only set the standards but also graded student submissions. In her spare time she cultivated benefactors, and when they died she reaped a harvest of bequests. She was indeed a model hospital administrator, nursing education director, and fund-raising dynamo.[15]

In 1921 the state legislature appropriated $25,000 for the care of indigent and crippled children. Miss Ariss was pleased to note that

> our hospital was one of three selected to do this work. The children come to us in the most deplorable condition of deformity. One boy, sixteen years

old, had never been able to walk since babyhood. His faithful dog pulled him on a sled and cart to school for years until he finished his grade work. Then the Orthopedic Commission made it possible for him to take six months treatment in the Hospital and the result is that this boy is now walking like other boys, taking a course in the Business College, and will soon be self-supporting.[16]

Ariss herself was a model of self-sufficiency. She led morning prayers for her charges, and when empty beds were available she prayed that the Lord would send in the suffering who needed care. "They seemed to come in from all directions after she prayed. . . . I didn't ever hear Miss Ariss pray that people would become sick but I did hear her pray that if people became ill, they would decide to come to our hospital." On his deathbed, Brother Van remarked to a nurse, actually Ariss's chosen successor, that he was fine because "Edith has fixed me up." The mortified Miss Lamb was astonished at his use of Miss Ariss's first name.[17]

The Nursing Apprenticeship

From the turn of the century (when the hospital was forced to close down temporarily for financial reasons) until America entered the Great War, Great Falls Deaconess was the site of all training for registered nurses in Montana. Fifty-eight nurses, most of them from outside the state, graduated during those years. Most did not have high school diplomas, although a few did have some experience in hospital work. Most were eighteen or nineteen years of age. Most also worked alongside lay trainees. As more vocational opportunities became available to them, few chose to don the habit and become Deaconesses. That did not imply that the religious impulse had disappeared, only that there were other ways of attaining grace.[18]

Many of that first generation of nursing graduates joined the Red Cross during the war and volunteered for duty overseas. When the influenza epidemic struck Montana there was a desperate shortage of trained nurses, and the Red Cross sent what assistance it could muster.[19] The second generation of Deaconesses was recruited from within the state, and the various units of the state's higher education system began to offer nursing education programs. During the 1920s, the colleges at Bozeman, Billings, and Havre became affiliated with Great Falls as training centers. Requirements differed from unit to unit, but generally applicants were required to be in good health, as certified by a physician. Each should bear a smallpox vaccination scar and have a certificate from a dentist indicating that her teeth were in good condition. Enlarged tonsils were to be removed.[20] This last is a nice piece of period medicine; tonsils were thought to be the locus of upper respiratory infections. Academically, applicants were expected to have at least two years of high school to meet state requirements, although the Bozeman college required a diploma. A suitable science background was important, and, of course, all candidates seeking entrance into the Deaconess schools of nursing had to be Protestant.

By the mid-1920s, Deaconess training was aimed at producing missionaries. Of the dozen or so for whom we have records, most went to the Far East. One woman journeyed to South Africa as a member of a Nazarene group. Each graduate had survived a difficult indoctrination. Novices rose at 5:30 A.M. and retired at 10:00 P.M. Their living conditions were spartan, and there were regular inspections of personal appearance and articles of clothing. Nurses were expected to remain quiet, not to laugh publicly, and to be physically fit: "The elevator will not be in use on Sundays unless in case of emergency, nor are the nurses allowed to use it on weekdays except when the duty of the hospital requires it."[21]

But their lives were not devoid of caring and good humor. Like young people everywhere, nursing students found ways to smooth over the rough edges of life: "Card playing and dancing were not permitted. We would be put out of school if we were caught doing either of these. Of course, many of us did break the rules without being caught. The Deaconesses were good sports and had a good sense of humor, in their special way. They were sort of other worldly."[22]

As the practice of medicine became more scientific, nursing practice also changed. Montana had no medical schools, and hence no interns to use as cheap labor, so nurses routinely took blood pressures, began intravenous procedures, and in general assumed tasks that might in other circumstances have been left to fledgling physicians. Obstetrics and pediatrics, traditional female concerns, were natural arenas for the expansion of nursing capabilities. Most of the material concerning precursors of nurse practitioning is anecdotal, but given Montana's weather, space, and isolation, the development of independent spirits would not be surprising.

Whether they were lay nurses or Deaconesses, the young women were surrounded by a paternalistic but caring community. White Cross Day each autumn coincided with the Thanksgiving harvest festivals. The Methodist churches of each district were asked to support offerings for each hospital. For example, in 1914 the Epworth League Methodist Episcopal of Dillon donated nine bath towels, two cloths, six bars of soap, sixteen quarts of fruit, and two glasses of jelly. As the state prospered, these annual affairs became more genteel. In Havre, the women of the Protestant churches held a tea and shower for the hospital. Prior to the tea the needs of the hospital were printed in the local newspaper. Ministers' wives poured, women's circles donated fancy baked goods, and the hospital offered tours of the facility. In towns with both Catholic and Deaconess hospitals, each group vied to have the first tea, to reap the greater dividends.[23]

The apprenticeship methods of the early Deaconess movement in Montana were suitable for the needs of the day. Because nursing was and is a profession with many avenues of development, however, it was not possible for the program to retain the level of faith and commitment to religious principles personified by Edith Augusta Ariss. The public health movement reached Montana just after the turn of the century with the establishment of the state Board of Health, which targeted spotted fever, silicosis/tuberculosis, immunization and quarantine programs, and hygiene instruction as areas needing nurses' participation. In addition, nurses could move into social service, which stressed different skills. The new scientific and public health–oriented medicine required more and better education for nurses.

Local nurses knew full well that the general tenor of the state education programs was poor. In 1932, some student nurses were assigned seventy hours per week of night duty; only five of the state's fourteen schools reported a forty-eight-hour week as normal for day work. Meeting professional standards and hospital budgetary requirements during the Great Depression was clearly impossible.[24] The somewhat tentative study of nursing education conducted by Josephine Goldmark in 1923 led to increased interest among nursing educators for some college affiliation in Montana.

College Nursing Programs

Montana nursing schools followed the Minnesota model, the first college-based three-year nursing program. During World War I (1914–18) the college at Bozeman offered emergency training for nurses, and in 1917–18 it established a regular nurses' training program. The college continued the program after the war, but no one enrolled between 1920 and 1923. The program for nurses in 1923 was a series of introductory courses, with chemistry, zoology, human physiology, bacteriology, dietetics, and something called "housewifery" forming the core for further training.[25]

The Great Depression severely curtailed higher education for nurses. As the New Deal health policy unfolded, hospitals became far less arenas for training nurses than sites for employing them. Changes in medical science—and in medical insurance—emphasized the need for college or university affiliation for training programs. In Montana, these difficulties were compounded by the old Deaconess nursing traditions and practices. How could a nursing program be melded into a nonsectarian public college and still retain the spiritual commitment of the original Deaconesses? The introduction of the associate's degree, which required fewer credits and less investment, further undermined the program. Hospital administrators strapped for cash preferred to hire nurses with an associate's degree, and the B.S. nursing certificate lost its value.[26]

Collegiate nursing programs concentrated on the problem of providing both academic and ward-based training. To raise the status of graduate nurses—the registered nurses of the future—and to meld hospital training programs with on-campus classes for a year, a five-year nursing degree was instituted. This term of study had become increasingly common in other professional areas such as engineering and architecture. It seemed an ideal solution. Hospitals would retain control of the clinical work, and the college would offer the cachet of a college degree. The college assumed the more expensive responsibility for instruction, and the hospital assigned the clinical workload. The arrangement was so successful that it is still in use today—much to the chagrin of university administrators who often bemoan the high cost of the nursing curriculum.[27] The college degree, however, had some unexpected consequences. Hospitals were suddenly faced with independent baccalaureate nurses who demanded both higher salaries and a certain degree of autonomy.[28]

Hospital Service versus University Education

The conflict between the demands of hospital service and university education is illustrated by a conflict that erupted in 1948 between the Montana State College (Bozeman) Nursing Program and Great Falls Deaconess Hospital. The argument exemplifies the complex new relationships between management, policy, and practice, in this case with a Deaconess student caught in the middle. The actors in the case were the director of nursing at Great Falls Deaconess, the president of the hospital's board of directors, and the hospital administrator and nursing students there; and, in Bozeman, Frank B. Cotner, the dean of the Division of Science (which included nursing), and Anna Pearl Sherrick, the director of the Montana State College Nursing Program.

The story begins with an agreement reached between the college and Great Falls Deaconess Hospital in 1937. The hospital agreed to provide young women with adequate living facilities, time to pursue an academic program, and clinical experience in a variety of specialties. The college, however, would have final approval on all instructors' credentials, and the dean of the Division of Science would be the final authority in instructional matters.

The agreement between the hospital and the college was updated in late May 1947. Montana State College (MSC) agreed to set standards for hospital training that met the criteria established by the Association of Graduate Schools of

Nursing Education. And when and if disciplinary problems arose, MSC would be the final authority.[29]

The problem surfaced in the spring of 1948 when a report from the nursing director at Great Falls sharply criticized the lack of coordination between the college curriculum at Bozeman and the clinical experience the students received in the hospital:

> It does not follow in the present curriculum setup that the teaching of disease or condition always covers the cases on the wards; for example, if in the course of study as now suggested, the Doctor is expected to discuss coronary heart disease, he would do so. The student may or may not see the coronary heart case until the next quarter. . . . Any number of diseases may be substituted for this illustration. . . . The medical lectures as scheduled are based upon the program used in medical schools.[30]

Dissatisfaction with the situation at Great Falls had been building, and discussions between the two groups had failed to resolve the matter. Now things escalated. In the autumn of 1948 Cotner wrote to the Great Falls administration: "It has come to the attention of MSC that the Montana Deaconess Hospital in Great Falls is interested in discontinuing the MSC nursing program. . . . Recently the School of Nursing, Campus Division, has found (1) the educational program for student nurses is below the standards of those set up in the working agreement, and (2) the quality of nursing service to be considerably below the standards proposed in the working agreement." In the view of MSC, these defects were primarily the result of "excessive night work." Great Falls responded: "It has been impossible to obtain enough student nurses to maintain our school of nursing."[31]

The controversy continued to develop and eventually involved the administrators in both cities. Great Falls wanted more students and less interference; Bozeman sought higher academic standards. In June 1950, C. K. Shiro, the administrator at Great Falls, announced that the hospital had fired its nursing director, Mathilde A. Haza. Haza was the third director to resign or be fired in the last five months. The chairman of the board, R. B. Richardson M.D., wrote to Dean Cotner, who was responsible for all science curricula at MSC, including nursing, that Director Haza had resigned. In his letter Richardson noted that Haza's "continued presence was extremely harmful to this institution. She was insubordinate and attempted to influence other members of the nursing staff. . . . Her influence with nursing students was also injurious. She made several derogatory statements regarding the administration of the hospital, the Chaplain of the hospital, the board of trustees and the medical staff."

There is no doubt that the Great Falls director had been a thorn. In a postscript to a letter complaining to her superiors, Haza aimed her darts at the MSC nursing program under the direction of Sherrick, which was in her view a program with little or no coordination: "There must be something wrong with Miss Sherrick's direction. Do you realize that she has lost all three directors of nursing [at Great Falls Deaconess] within five months? As far as I can see, a director must be a puppet in her hands and any sign of independent thinking is frowned upon. She is a dictator and no one else knows or understands school administration."[32]

When two MSC students at Great Falls organized an attempt to save Haza's job, retribution was swift. After the new college term had begun in the fall and students were properly enrolled for their work at Great Falls, the new director of nursing expelled the "ringleader" of the revolt, Miss Marjorie Merriman. The list of Merriman's infractions included "improper uniform, smoking in full uniform, meandering late to morning chapel, a nonchalant, unconcerned attitude, staying up until 2:00 A.M. or all hours, rudeness and having a pinkish trend."[33]

Miss Merriman had a formidable ally, however. Her mother organized a counterattack focused on Dean Cotner, who began to receive complaints from all sides. The nurses to a woman signed a protest of the treatment of their ringleader and resigned. Another group of nurses, in the same class but serving in the mental health facility in Warm Springs, joined the protest and asked MSC what it was doing to remedy the situation. Later that fall, the minister at the First Methodist Church in Great Falls wrote to Cotner urging him to resolve the situation: "We are interested in the hospital and we are interested in the girls and their continuing in a great profession based on the desire to serve in a Christian way."[34]

The involvement of the church, which had the ultimate authority over the hospital, was not good news for nursing students. In November 1950, J. Homer Magee, the superintendent of the Glacier Park District of the Methodist church, wrote to Cotner:

> I have been very much interested in this Deaconess Hospital mess because I have some responsibility for the church but have not felt that I could rush into things until my position was recognized. . . . The trouble started, as you know, when the new director of nurses inaugurated new rules and with it a gag rule that is still in force. The administration has adopted a policy of picking scapegoats. . . . When the trouble did not subside the chaplain was made the next scapegoat, and to save his future I had to work out a resignation and terminal leave. The accusations against him are unfounded.[35]

More retaliation against the scapegoats was forthcoming. Dean Cotner received a letter from the Great Falls students informing him that their student council had been dissolved although "all other units have one," the nursing honorary society had been banned, permission to visit the chaplain would now be given only for spiritual matters, chapel would be used for roll call inspection, there would be no more allowance of time for married students living off campus, and senior nurses caring for private patients would no longer receive the customary $5 fee. Furthermore, they wrote, "we students are not receiving a proper education," and they reminded the dean that "we have had a choice of nine nursing centers." The Great Falls MSC program was in imminent danger of collapse.

Mr. Magee wrote again five days later: "My best information is that there will be quite a few girls lost to nursing unless they are allowed to transfer to other schools. Because this business is a lot deeper than a few rules."[36] Cotner responded that he would arrange a transfer of the entire group to another college and temporarily suspend the agreement with Great Falls. Magee agreed, and noted that the real fly in the ointment was the hospital administrator, who told the board and church one thing, the nurses another, and the school quite another.

In the end, a classic bureaucratic solution was found. Miss Merriman (the ringleader), her family, her support group in Great Falls, the hospital, and MSC officials all breathed a sigh of relief when a budgetary review revealed a surplus of just enough cash to allow Miss Merriman to transfer and enroll in the program at Billings.[37] The surplus was only $50, but the transfer was a workable solution.

This story illustrates some of the difficulties facing nursing education in the first half of the twentieth century. New science and technology drove curricular concerns in higher education while increasing secularization and economic opportunity created a nursing environment quite different from the one Methodist hospital administrators expected. Without a teaching hospital, a college or university had to rely on cooperative institutions. In turn, the largely religious foundations on which hospitals were grounded found it difficult to accommodate student nurses' changing mores and expectations.

Although the period of frontier nursing embraced only two, or perhaps three, generations, the legacy of that frontier experience is still discernible. Sparsely populated Montana has as much frontier today as it had in the time of Frederick Jackson Turner. Physician's assistants and nurse practitioners fill gaps left in local practice, and rural health care continues to be an intractable problem. Furthermore, local communities no longer support rural hospitals and nurses as they did in the first half of the century. After 1960, many of the small rural hospitals closed, in some instances replaced by medical assistance facilities. The feeling of isolation one might expect to associate with a turn-of-the-century frontier experience became actually more intense rather than less so.

"There is nobody but me here and this is different. You don't get experience from others around you—another person might have different experience or more experience and you learn from others. I miss that a lot."[38] Nurses could read journals, of course, but none seemed really pertinent to rural or frontier nursing.

Frontier conditions demanded great sacrifice from all women engaged in medical work: physicians, nurses, and assistants. Establishing and maintaining nursing education programs was difficult when populations were impermanent. In the absence of trained nurses, student nurses were under great pressure to work rather than to learn and observe. The ideals of educators and nursing professionals were not shared by Methodist hospital administrators, who were concerned more about the moral climate and staffing issues than the quality of the education given to students. At the same time, all parties agreed that, following the models of Nightingale and Fliedner, nursing's foundations were as much spiritual as practical. In this sense the historical basis of nursing in the West offers a valuable perspective for considering contemporary nursing concerns.

8 Chinese Medicine on the "Gold Mountain"

Tradition, Adaptation, and Change

PAUL D. BUELL

The "Gold Mountain"

Chinese and American societies are often characterized as worlds apart and utterly different, the one a staid Old World culture changing only very slowly, the other the dynamic product of a moving frontier, a cultural and ethnic melting pot. In fact, the contrast is inaccurate; the United States has stronger roots in European history than Americans are often willing to admit, and China has exhibited far more dynamism in its long history than is often recognized. The China of today, for example, would have been barely recognizable as recently as five hundred years ago, before the high population density that we associate with China today first developed. Go back a thousand years and there was no tea drinking and little rice growing. Even the presently used Chinese writing system is only a little more than two thousand years old, instituted when the unifier Ch'in Shih-huang-ti and others helped to standardize written Chinese.

China has also had its own "moving frontier" and is even more a melting pot than the United States. The Chinese society of the present is the end result of the assimilation of non-Chinese cultures over the centuries. The earliest China was located along the Yellow River valley. By the fourth century B.C. it was well on the way to incorporating the cultures of the Yang-tzu and Szu-ch'uan. First contacts with the extreme south came under the Ch'in and Han (255 B.C.–A.D. 220), and by T'ang times (A.D. 618–906) coastal areas and some interior strategic routes were becoming Sinicized. The southwest was added under the Ming (1368–1644) and Ch'ing (1644–1911) Dynasties, Inner Mongolia and Hsin-chiang in the nineteenth century, and Tibet in the twentieth.

This process has continued with Chinese overseas colonization, primarily accomplished through the societies of the Canton Delta region, at first of the islands and nations immediately surrounding China, and then in the more distant New World, called by the Chinese "Gold Mountain," land of opportunities. In the American West, the moving frontier of the Gold Mountain encountered the moving frontier of the United States. There, Americans coming from the East first encountered the Chinese, and the Chinese the Americans, in an interaction that continues today.

Chinese Emigration

Chinese migration to the United States began with the annexation of California (taken from Mexico) and the discovery of gold there. Chinese laborers from those counties of Kuang-tung Province that were situated around the Pearl River estuary (Canton Delta) appeared almost everywhere in the gold fields and in the coastal towns supporting the gold fields, especially San Francisco. They performed almost every task, including mining, which they were often better at than Western miners thanks to superior Cantonese technology. The Chinese prospered and began sending a large part of their wealth home to support their families and to pay the passage of their clansmen to the new frontier. California indeed became a "Gold Mountain," a paradise for Chinese immigrants and an attractive investment for the Canton Delta economic elite. Chinese merchants and other commercial entrepreneurs of every sort appeared more or less simultaneously with the first Chinese laborers and miners, and soon became key parts of Gold Mountain society.[1]

Among the merchant emigrants were traditional Chinese doctor-pharmacists, a merchant class well represented throughout the Canton Delta, particularly in Hsiang-shan County, with its great medical schools, large pharmacies, and even charity clinics. Through these merchant doctors, herbal medicine,[2] the most important of all Chinese medical traditions, was widely available in the Chinese and non-Chinese communities of the "Gold Mountain" frontier. Merchant doctors also brought with them other traditions of healing, including traditional bone setting and even moxacautery, the practice whereby a prepared *Artemisia* is burned at certain points on the body to stimulate the flow of healing forces.[3] Most of the other traditions of Chinese medicine were represented as well and practiced by amateur healers, including dietary therapy,[4] shamanic intervention and faith healing, and even magic.[5]

Chinese Medicine

Although there is now a substantial literature on traditional Chinese medicine as practiced in the New World, a great deal of confusion remains. This is largely due to mistaken comparisons between what is seen as a unified tradition of Western, cosmopolitan medicine and a Chinese medicine that is quite different. In fact, there has never been a single unified tradition of Chinese medicine; rather, reinforcing streams of development have existed ranging from purely magical and spiritual methods to theoretical appreciations as complicated as any employed in the West.[6] Each stream developed in response to particular Chinese conditions and health needs and according to cultural assumptions that have evolved considerably over time. Like China itself, which has had periods of unity and disunity, China's various medical traditions and systems have at times shared cultural and theoretical assumptions that have drawn them together, only to go more or less separate ways when circumstances changed. In addition, there has always been a tension between local and national traditions in China, and also between the values of the elite (associated with national regimes and ideologies) and the practices of the masses. As a rule, the more a medical system was associated with the elite, and thus with the court, the greater its foundation in written theory; the more popular, the more pragmatic was its approach and the greater was the tendency to make theory align with facts.

The most sophisticated medical traditions of China, including acupuncture and herbal medicine, were the last to develop as organized systems. Nevertheless, both have strong roots in earlier practices, much as modern Western medicine still displays vestiges of the humoral medicine from which it developed. In part, the late development of acupuncture and herbal medicine is a reflection of technology. There could be, for example, no acupuncture before the development of fine steel needles, which occurred sometime at the beginning of the Christian era. Likewise, modern herbal medicine owes a great deal to printing, which allowed the dissemination and systemization of lore garnered over the centuries. Ideology and the creation of elite intellectual traditions that sought to dictate national values played roles as well.

It was once widely believed that most illness arose as a result of conflict or disharmony between the living and the spirits of the dead, and the most ancient forms of Chinese medicine involved various methods of manipulating the spirit world. Natural forces, including "evil wind" (*feng*), the ultimate environmental explanation for otherwise unexplained illness and still an important facet of Chinese medical theory, could also cause illness and had likewise to be propitiated.

Also very old in Chinese medicine, and intimately associated with the very idea of the physician in China, is the belief in the special powers of the shaman to deal with the menaces of the spiritual world personified as "demons."[7] This "demonic" tradition of Chinese medicine included not only the mystic séance of the shaman to fetch (if possible) the errant soul of the patient, but also the use of pressure, heat, or some physical object to drive out or control the demons congregating within. As this tradition became systematized, moxacautery and massage became preferred forms of treatment. Later, acupuncture appeared. One early form employed metal implements reminiscent of the ritual dagger of the Eurasian shaman, strongly expressing the roots of acupuncture in shamanic practice and "demonic" medicine. Ultimately acupuncture became the dominant practice, and classical books originally written for massage and moxacautery were rewritten with acupuncture in mind. The result was China's first consistent theoretical medical literature, the texts making up the *Yellow Emperor's Inner Classic.*

During the same period that demonic medicine was being systematized and transformed, herbal medicine was becoming increasingly important. As it is now practiced, Chinese herbal medicine owes a great deal to the experiments and theorizing of Chinese alchemists of the last centuries B.C. They sought to utilize drugs, foods, and herbs to purify the body and free the spirit from the dross of material existence as preparation for immortality. To this end they tried to classify substances and their effects. By the fourth century A.D. their experiences, along with traditional herbal lore, had been codified into the first documents of the Chinese herbal literature, the *pen-ts'ao.*[8]

Thus, by the first centuries of the Christian era, most of the components of Chinese medicine as it is now practiced were already present, although in some cases in rudimentary form. What has taken place since has been the creation and expansion of a theoretical base only hinted at in the most ancient traditions, the accumulation of still more pragmatic experience, and the enrichment of Chinese traditions through foreign influences.

The greatest theoretical advances were made during Han times, which saw the first efforts to create not only a unified medical theory, but also a whole philosophical basis for the subsequent development of Chinese thought and ideology. The men of the Han Dynasty and their intellectual successors increasingly sought rational, mechanistic, and mathematical explanations of the phenomena of the universe, including medicine and healing, while downplaying the role of ancestral spirits and demonic and magical elements. In so doing they built on foundations laid down by Chinese thinkers of earlier centuries.

Key components of this reinterpretation of the physical and spiritual universe were the concepts of *yin* and *yang*, the female and male principles, out of which everything was believed to have developed. Mixtures of *yin* and *yang* with various properties yielded the "five transitional phases," the Chinese elements. Also an important part of the system was a belief in *ch'i*, the energy or "vapor" that permeates the universe and is the means by which *yin, yang,* and the five elements can be conceived of as a dynamic system.

It took the Chinese centuries to work out all the details of this new world-view and apply it to medicine. Later, under the direct influence of Indian philosophy as mediated by Buddhism, a materialist metaphysics was added, resulting in the complicated philosophical system known as Neoconfucianism. From the twelfth century onward, this philosophy permeated all aspects of Chinese life, including medicine.

Acupuncture was the first medical practice to be reworked in the new mold. A rationalist, materialist view is already implicit in the texts of the *Yellow Emperor's Inner Classic,* which reinterpret the organs of the body in terms of a complex system that associates organs and other physical systems with *yin, yang,* the five transitional phases, and *ch'i.* Gone are most, but not all, of the demons of earlier tradition. In the new view, acupuncture needles were inserted not to drive out assemblies of evil spirits causing harm, but to direct *ch'i* (*yin ch'i*), to restore balance within a mechanistic bodily system that had somehow become unbalanced by environmental or other elements. Diagnosis was also in terms of *yin, yang,* the five transitional phases, and *ch'i* and became increasingly sophisticated as time passed. Acupuncture practices, and, later, herbal medicine, came to view illness not as due to a single pathology or dysfunction but as a reflection of cooperating causes and effects, including some generated by the treatment itself, a possible cause of further imbalances in an already unbalanced system. This view of illness is fundamental to almost all forms of Chinese medicine and is one of the major differences between Chinese medicine and Western cosmopolitan medicine.

Even as acupuncture was changing to reflect new theoretical considerations, herbal medicine was changing under the influence of acupuncture theory and Neoconfucianism. The change was in large part accomplished through increasingly sophisticated systems for classifying herbs and their therapeutic effects. By China's early medieval period (fifth and sixth centuries) at the latest, herbs were being classified not only in terms of their medicinal effects and ability to promote Taoist physiological alchemy, but also by taste, by how they interacted with other herbs in compounds, and by whether they were extremely heating, cooling, moderately heating or cooling, or neutral according to a system probably borrowed from India. By late medieval times, specific properties of herbs were being associated with specific conditions and disease syndromes, as the following examples from the fourteenth-century dietary manual *Yin-shan cheng-yao,* compiled by Hu Szu-hui for the then Mongol emperors of China, indicate.[9] "Leaking dysentery," by the way, is dysentery that allows vital force in the form of *ch'i* to "leak out." "Evil heat" is heat as a pathological agent and is countered by the cooling qualities of foxtail millet. Note the appeal to authority in the form of a quotation from an earlier *pen-ts'ao:*

Foxtail millet is salty in flavor, slightly cooling and lacks poison [i.e., has no strong medicinal effect]. It is good for nourishing kidney *ch'i*. It removes [evil] heat of spleen and stomach. It increases *ch'i*. Old [foxtail millet] is best. It is used to regulate [evil] heat of the stomach, and excessive thirst. It benefits urination and controls leaking dysentery. The *T'ang-pen chu* says: "There are many varieties of foxtail millets. The kernels are fine like *liang-mi* [millet]. The uniform washed grains obtained from fine millet; are *che-mi*." [3, 1B]

By the thirteenth and fourteenth centuries, acupuncture and herbal medicine had finally been unified under the umbrella of correspondence medicine, the only medical theory in Chinese history to place these two disparate forms of practice on the same theoretical basis. Similarly, a related Neoconfucianism, which also expressed itself in terms of complex relationships of *yin, yang,* the five phases, and flows of *ch'i* governed by archetypal principles (*li*) expressive of a universal *tao,* dominated Chinese philosophy and ideology. In the case of acupuncture, correspondence theory worked very well and, after a great deal of fine-tuning, is still followed today. Herbal medicine, which continued to assimilate massive amounts of empirical data not easily explained by correspondence medicine theory, was another matter entirely.

There were thousands upon thousands of herbs in use, many nationally but most only locally. Only a few books even attempted to list them all, none successfully because new remedies were constantly being discovered. Given China's lack of systematic botanical and faunal classification, it was almost impossible to ensure that the same herb was always referred to by the same name.

Although correspondence theory was progressively developed by medical theoreticians over the next centuries, it became more and more an erudite exercise ill suited to the vast pragmatic reality that was Chinese traditional medicine. While some traditions, including moxacautery and acupressure massage, and to a limited extent exercise, could accommodate themselves to correspondence medicine through their association with acupuncture theory, other traditions remained outside the pale entirely. Shamanic cures and much of Chinese folk psychology, for example, have never lost their demons.

By the eighteenth century, herbal medicine and many other traditions that constituted the real mainstream of medical development in China were being practiced in a way that was increasingly at variance with theory, leading, in some cases, to a massive reexamination of theory itself. In fact, even before the introduction of Western cosmopolitan medicine, the Chinese themselves were challenging many of the fundamental assumptions of their past medical traditions. For the first time in many centuries, efforts were made to create entirely new theories.[10] The human body, for example, was looked at as it actually was rather than as the construct of the acupuncturists. There were still no dissections, but at least one Chinese doctor participated as an observer at executions by "slow slicing." The internal organs of the victim were there for all to see, and they were not as correspondence theory held them to be.[11]

Such was the intellectual and medical environment when Chinese medicine was first brought to America. Theory, though acknowledged, was often ignored in practice as something, in the words of Seattle pharmacist Hen Sen Chin, too subtle to understand. When theory was considered, it was frequently reworked to accommodate new facts and observed reality. The contrast between what was said and what was done was made all the more striking by the failure of acupuncture, the tradition in Chinese medicine best supported by theory, to become established on the American frontier. In the nineteenth century, acupuncture was still associated with the elite, and therefore was not popular among the peasant and merchant cultures that produced nearly all the immigrants to the Gold Mountain.

Chinese Medicine in America

Chinese medicine came to California with the earliest immigrants and moved along with them into the interior. By the late 1860s it was a general phenomenon in the frontier West. At that time, Chinese society in America was located mainly in interior mining communities and work camps, although the cities on the West Coast also had large populations of Chinese. It was only with the end of the various gold and silver rushes in the West and the imposition of anti-Chinese immigration quotas that the Chinese colonization tide flowed backward, into the larger cities where Chinese communities were too strong to be uprooted.

From the very beginning, Chinese medical practitioners working on the Gold Mountain served two clienteles: the Chinese themselves and an increasingly large number of non-Chinese residents. The popularity of Chinese medicine among the latter group may have been due either to the unavailability of Western cosmopolitan medicine in frontier communities or to frustration with Western medicine as it was then practiced. Chinese medicine's different attitude toward patients, women in particular, may also have helped to attract non-Chinese patients.[12] Chinese doctors and even amateur practitioners, as we shall see, adapted themselves quickly to new conditions, just as they had done in China over the centuries. It was, above all, the ability of Chinese medical practitioners to relate to the non-Chinese community and the perceived usefulness of Chinese medicine as a part of the local health care system that helped preserve Chinese medicine after the mining and labor camps began to close and the Chinese themselves became a persecuted minority. During the difficult years of the early twentieth century, in fact, Chinese medicine survived as an organized system largely by serving the white community.

We are fortunate to possess a rich variety of sources with which to write a history of traditional Chinese medicine in the United States. Americans can thus come to understand an important aspect of their own historical and cultural development and also glimpse several important aspects of Chinese medicine that would be less apparent in a purely Chinese environment. The sources include an abundance of photographs, early newspaper reports, travelogues written by persons who visited the gold and silver fields and other early frontier communities, oral histories, and, most important, surviving collections of herbs, recipe books, and other materials from Chinese apothecaries who once operated in settlements as far afield as Boise, Idaho; John Day, Oregon; Seattle, Washington; and Vancouver, British Columbia. From Seattle comes a remarkable recipe book, the handwritten *Yao-fang,* a compilation of the accumulated medical knowledge of Seattle's early Chinese community.[13] Since there is far too much material to review in detail, I will confine myself to a few general observations.

Adherence to Tradition

Perhaps the most striking aspect of Chinese medicine as it has been practiced in the United States is its faithfulness to Chinese tradition and to a larger Chinese cultural and intellectual environment. Wolfram Eberhard pointed out some decades ago, when studying the documentary and other remains of a Chinese temple in Marysville, California, the degree to which that temple, even though clearly resident on the Gold Mountain, remained completely a part of China, an extension of a greater Chinese civilization of which it was a part.[14] The Chinese medicine of the Gold Mountain was no different. Although local *materiae medicae* were incorporated into Gold Mountain recipe books and formularies, Chinese doctors in the New World remained remarkably loyal to the herbs and formulas in use in their homeland and continued to produce complex, well-balanced recipes fully in accord with traditional Chinese diagnostic principles, as the two examples below show. The first, a hangover remedy, is from the *Yin-shan cheng-yao;* the second, a cure for gonorrhea, is from the *Yao-fang.*

   1. Detoxifying Dried Orange Peel Puree
   It is used to cure intoxication that persists, vomiting and bile in the throat.
   [Prepared] fragrant orange [*Citrus sinensis*] peel
       (one *chin;* remove the white)
   Prepared mandarin orange peel (one *chin;* remove the white)
   Sandalwood (four *liang*)

Kudzu flower (one-half *chin*)
Mungbean flower (one-half *chin*)
Ginseng (two *liang;* remove the green shoots)
Cardamom kernel (two *liang*)
Salt (six *liang;* roast)
   Make a fine powder of ingredients. Each day take a little in boiling water on an empty stomach. [2, 5A]

2. Recipe for When Gonorrhea First Appears and Is Very Painful
Dried, whole *Buthus martensi*—12 *ch'ien*
Processed scale of pangolin, *Manis pentadactyla*—4 *ch'ien*
Bark of Amur cork tree, *Phellodendron sp.*—4 *ch'ien*
Receptacle or seed of the lotus, *Nelumbo nucifera*—4 *ch'ien*
Rhizome of *Aniemarrhena asphodeloides*—4 *ch'ien*
Root of Baical skullcap, *Scutellaria baicalensis*—1 *ch'ien*
Sclerotium of *Polyporus umbellatus*—4 *ch'ien*
Myrrh—4 *ch'ien*
Talc—4 *ch'ien*
Herb of *Saposhnikovia divaricata*—2 *ch'ien*
Herb or flower of *Schizonepeta tenuifolia*—13 *ch'ien*
Rhizome of woolly grass, *Imperata cylindrica*—4 *ch'ien*
Fruit of the honeysuckle, *Lonicera japonica*—6 *ch'ien*
Rhizome of water plantain, *Alisma plantago-aquatica*—4 *ch'ien*
Frankincense—3 *ch'ien*
Liquorice "bud"—23 *ch'ien*
Herb and seed of the fern, *Lygodium sp.*—2 *ch'ien*
[text partly unreadable]
   If ulcers appear, add:
Safflower, *Carthamus tinctorius*
End of the lateral root of *Angelica sinensis*.[15]

The first recipe is carefully balanced in terms of the values associated with Chinese herbs, but like most time-honored hangover concoctions it seeks primarily to restore the body's electrolyte and fluid balances. It concocts a fine medicinal powder of a type popular in Islamic medicine, perhaps its remote origin, but also common to the Chinese tradition. The second, by no means the most complex recipe to survive from an American source, was to be taken as a *chi,* a traditional Chinese dose, with the herbs finely ground and combined, then boiled in water for drinking. Although this was the typical method for consuming herbs, "pills" were also used, taken orally or dissolved in the mouth. There was also at hand a vast assortment of suppositories.
   Another sign of a quite traditional approach to Chinese medicine on the part

of its American practitioners is the continued use of traditional Chinese works as reference materials. The Ah-fong apothecary of Boise, Idaho,[16] for example, appears to have had a large library of herbals and similar works, including the *T'ang-yeh pen-ts'ao,* by Wang Hao-ku,[17] a mid-thirteenth-century work widely used in China and an important theoretical appreciation of correspondence medicine. The same was true of other pharmacies, judging by the material that survives. Another feature common to traditional Chinese pharmacies in America was the handwritten recipe books handed down from father to son and in most cases originally compiled in China sometime in the nineteenth century. Seattle's Wing Luke Asian Museum has a number of examples once used by Seattle's early Chinese doctors and contributed to the museum's Chinese medicine collection by Hen Sen Chin.

Adaptation to a New Environment

While Chinese physicians practicing in the New World remained remarkably loyal to their inherited traditions, a second noteworthy feature of their practice was the degree to which they adapted their practices to their new environment. The disease environment of the New World was different from that of China. In particular, the Chinese encountered new diseases, including occupational diseases such as mercury poisoning associated with mining. The population served by Chinese doctors in the Gold Mountain was also different demographically: it was younger, at least initially, and tended more to be male than female.

The recipe from the *Yao-fang* quoted above exemplifies the kinds of differences noticeable between a traditional Chinese medical practice in China and one in the New World. Gonorrhea was not unknown in Kuang-tung Province, but it was clearly a great deal more prevalent among the Chinese in America, at least judging by the number of recipes for treating this and other venereal diseases in traditional recipe books. Also more prevalent among the Gold Mountain Chinese were traumatic injuries, due, perhaps, to a more rough-and-tumble life-style. The *Yao-fang* was used and added to from the 1860s down to the 1970s, and the types of recipes it contains are probably a good indication of the epidemiology of Seattle's Chinese community, and, indirectly, of the non-Chinese patients treated by Chinese doctors. Major recipe categories in the *Yao-fang* (out of 166 recipes) include the following:

1. Venereal diseases (perhaps one-fifth of the recipes)
2. Traumatic injury (13 recipes)
3. Respiratory complaints (13 recipes)

4. Problems of the gastrointestinal tract and digestive complaints (12 recipes)
5. Tonics (10 recipes)
6. Antismoking or opium addiction (10 recipes)
7. Eye, ear, and throat (9 recipes)

Other important categories are eye, skin, and teeth recipes and herbal treatments for rheumatism and other common complaints.[18] The surviving recipe books and other documents preserving recipes and disease categories also provide evidence of efforts by Chinese doctors serving the Gold Mountain to innovate—to experiment in the hopes of finding new cures for old diseases, and for new ones.

C. K. Ah-fong, for example, although he was following very good Chinese precedent, seems to have made an effort to collect rattlesnakes, which he is said to have thrust alive into the purest alcohol he could find. The resulting "rattlesnake wine," or tincture of rattlesnake, is said to have worked well for arthritis and to have been a painful but effective cure for impotency.[19] In the latter case the tincture worked by contracting and tightening flaccid tissue, in the former by reducing swelling. C. K. Ah-fong also seems to have experimented with various herbs and other substances (it must be remembered that Chinese herbal medicine is by no means confined to herbs) to cure mercury poisoning, unfortunately without success.[20] Other Chinese doctors had special cures as well. A contemporary practitioner, Seattle's Hen Sen, has even made an effort to revive *hsien,* the moxa-laden stones that were a primitive form of acupuncture therapy in early times. He is also known for adapting his herbal cures to accord with the diet of his Gold Mountain clients, including the chemical residues found in their foods.

I could assemble numerous examples of what appears to be assimilation on the part of traditional Chinese doctors, but how much assimilation actually occurred? The rattlesnake is a New World reptile, but the practice of putting snakes and other creatures and substances into alcohol to produce a tincture for later use had been well established in Chinese practice for centuries. The fourteenth-century *Yin-shan cheng-yao* (3, 5B–6B), for example, from which I quoted above, mentions the following medical tinctures: tiger bone liquor (i.e., tincture of ground, roasted tiger bone); wolfthorn berry (*Lycium chinense*) liquor; Chinese foxglove liquor; pine knot liquor (tincture of ground, boiled pine knots, "collected on the fifth day of the fifth month"); China root (*Poria cocos*) liquor; pine root liquor; tincture of pine root sap; lamb liquor; tincture of mutton; *Acanthopanax* bark liquor; and *castoreum,* a tincture of the ground penis and testes of the seals *Callorhinus ursinus* or *Phoca vitulina*. Cures for heavy metal poisoning are also nothing new to Chinese medicine; Taoists and others regularly poisoned themselves with arsenic and other heavy metals to promote a brief appearance of renewed youth and potency. Hen Sen's innovations also make good sense traditionally. His *hsien* are an innovation only in that they had not been used in thousands of years and no one was quite sure what a *hsien* was or how it was used. Alteration of recipes to suit dietary peculiarities is also nothing new. The practice was already well established in the *Yin-shan cheng-yao*, whose author was particularly concerned about the alcoholism and overindulgence of his Mongol masters.

Chinese Medicine in a New Era

The decline of America's Chinese communities in the late nineteenth and early twentieth centuries due to Chinese exclusion severely affected not only the Chinese communities themselves but also the practice of traditional Chinese medicine in America. Many pharmacies simply went out of business, a process hastened by the difficulty of obtaining supplies of traditional herbs due to endemic warfare in China and on the surrounding seas during the 1930s and 1940s.[21] Pharmacies had to change to survive. Most often the changes did not violate the traditions of Chinese medicine. Sometimes, however, more drastic changes were necessary, changes that radically altered the character of the medicine being practiced.

Among the Chinese practices continuing to adhere to a more or less traditional medicine in the new era was that of the Ah-fong family in Idaho. C. K. Ah-fong, the founder of the practice and its head into the 1920s, physically moved his practice as times changed and consciously sought a new clientele as the Idaho Chinese community declined around him. When C. K. Ah-fong first opened his Idaho practice, in 1866, it was in the mining town of Atlanta, then a focus of Idaho development. There he treated a mixed but predominantly young male community. Common complaints were traumatic injury, industrial diseases including mercury poisoning, and the ravages of venereal disease and heavy drinking. He treated his patients successfully, or so his contemporaries thought, but when the mining industry declined toward the end of the century, Ah-fong's practice in Atlanta was no longer viable. Consequently, in 1889, C. K. Ah-fong moved his practice and his family to Boise, by then the new center of Idaho development. There he found a population that was still largely mixed, although Chinese numbers declined rapidly after the turn of the century, and young, although less so than Atlanta's. It also included large numbers of women and even a few old people, more as time passed.[22] Boise's population was thus better balanced demographically and socially than Atlanta's, and its complaints were typical of any American city of comparable size containing reasonable proportions of the sexes and representatives of most age groups. Traumatic injuries still occurred, although in lesser numbers, and there were far fewer industrial diseases; prostitution and drinking continued to take their toll. Most common, judging from surviving documents, were respiratory problems, arthritis, gout, skin, and female complaints. C. K. Ah-fong was particularly successful in this last regard. The Western medicine of the time was not very responsive to female patients, whose conditions were often considered imaginary by Western doctors. The contrasting attitude of Chinese medicine made Chinese doctors attractive to Boise's female community, who, according to Ah-fong family and local tradition, became major customers of the practice.

Thus, by moving to Boise, C. K. Ah-fong was able to find new customers to compensate for those he had lost in Atlanta when mining declined. In spite of the new environment, the Ah-fongs, whatever their clientele and whatever its complaints, continued to practice a traditional medicine that was almost identical, rattlesnakes aside, to that found in the Canton Delta in the nineteenth century. This continued into the 1960s, when Gerald Ah-fong finally closed the practice and retired. In only one significant respect did the Ah-fongs accommodate themselves to the Gold Mountain—namely, in the area of licensure.

Although initially intended to eliminate incompetent physicians from the ranks of Western doctors, licensure was also, in the era of Chinese exclusion, used against traditional Chinese doctors. By Idaho law, all those practicing before a certain date were to be licensed as physicians, whatever their training. When the measure was not applied to him, C. K. Ah-fong sued and became one of the few traditional Chinese practitioners ever to be recognized as an M.D.[23]

Although his M.D. was unusual, otherwise C. K. Ah-fong's experience was repeated elsewhere in the early West. The John Day Lung On–Ing Hay practice was much like Ah-fong's except that its territory was largely rural.[24] Like the Ah-fongs, Lung On and Ing Hay had a largely white clientele but continued to practice a more or less traditional medicine. The same seems to have been true of early Seattle practitioners, with Hen Sen's own highly conservative approach continuing what has now become a tradition extending over a century. Vancouver has also remained a bastion of Chinese traditional medicine, as materials from a pharmacy studied by Nancy Turner and her colleagues make clear.[25] Only a short time ago there were still more or less traditional herb shops in Vancouver's Chinatown, one of the largest Chinese communities in North America. At one of them I observed a highly conservative arrangement whereby a doctor pronounced diagnoses separately from the druggist who made up the prescriptions, as in the great pharmacies of old China. Unlike those of Boise and John Day, however, Vancouver's Chinese doctors have continued to serve a largely Chinese clientele, perhaps making some of the accommodations observed elsewhere unnecessary.

Nonetheless, for all the conservatism and persistence of traditionalism in Chinese medicine, there have been compromises too. One major change, here and abroad (particularly in Taiwan and Hong Kong), has been the recent tendency for Chinese medicine to take up Western manufactured medicines, including, where legal, antibiotics.[26] Diagnosis has also changed. Although specific techniques and practices have varied considerably from one practitioner to another, and from one medical system to another, traditional Chinese diagnosis avoided simplistic characterizations of a given syndrome, looking instead at underlying patterns and root causes. Most diagnoses were formulated not only in terms of specific symptoms—"signs" (*hou*) and "physical manifestations" of disease (*hsing*)—but also in terms of what Paul Unschuld calls "pathoconditions" (*cheng*),[27] fundamental dysfunctions below the surface that may even run counter to apparent symptoms. In using herbs to treat illness, a Chinese doctor had to take all of these different indications—signs, physical manifestations, and pathoconditions—into consideration to formulate a prescription and perhaps other associated treatment as well. Furthermore, his prescriptions aimed not only to treat all evident and underlying conditions, but also to compensate for any side effects of the medicines themselves.

Formulas were often arrived at through consulting traditional reference works for a "base formula" that was intended to treat the syndrome in general terms.[28] The base formula was then fine-tuned with additional herbs to reflect the specific diagnosis, which could differ in important details from the general syndrome or could be complicated by other patterns not related to the general syndrome, including the physical characteristics and even the life-style of the patient.

Such diagnosis was not only difficult to do, especially for practitioners whose grounding in theory was weak, it was often incomprehensible to patients. Nowadays, simpler categories are often employed, many borrowed from the terminology of Western cosmopolitan medicine. Rarer now are references to "wounded middle burner" or "*yang-ch'i* degeneration," perhaps complicated by "invasion of cold evil," as parts of a complicated diagnosis. More common today are discussions of cancer, a disease syndrome that does not even exist in traditional Chinese medicine, and Parkinson's disease. Similarly, many herbalists practicing in this country, aware that their non-Chinese or assimilated clientele probably does not appreciate the subtleties of traditional Chinese fine-tuning of formulas, have simplified their formulas, leaving out expensive or hard-to-get herbs. Since this has been done in China as well, herbalists practicing in this country may simply be following a larger trend. It is also true that many herbalists today simply do not know how to do things the old way and have no choice but to practice a simplified form of traditional medicine.

Nonetheless, for all the apparent abasement, traditional Chinese forces may still be at work in the use of Western drugs and the simplified diagnoses. It is clear, for example, that the Chinese have for centuries accepted new remedies not yet fully assimilated into the tradition, before their properties have been worked out in detail. The *Yin-shan cheng-yao,* for example, includes new medicinal foods to which Hu Szu-hui assigned medical value even though he was uncertain of their precise application (e.g., wolf meat). The same text also includes straight borrowings from traditional Mongolian and even Muslim medicine. Is the sudden incorporation of antibiotics so different? Moreover, folk diagnosis of illness has never been as sophisticated as that practiced by professional doctors. Given all-too-simple categories such as demon possession and *ku* poisoning, why not use cancer or Parkinson's disease too? Even the use of simplified formulas to respond to a simplified view of illness may have traditional Chinese precedents. Not all Chinese doctors were *ming-i,* "famous doctors" known far and wide for their effective cures and ability to put together formulas with one hundred or more herbs on the spot. There have always been less qualified practitioners doing the best they could with what they had at hand.

In conclusion, the interactions of Chinese and Western medicines and the history of Chinese practitioners on the Gold Mountain stand as yet another chapter in the ongoing, centuries-old expansion of Chinese medicine and culture. From the perspective of Chinese immigrants, the mountain West became a new Chinese frontier, a place where ancient traditions, including medical and pharmaceutical theories and practices, could flourish and continue to evolve.

Introduction

1. Elizabeth Raymond, "Middle Ground and Marginal Space: Sense of Place in the Middle West and the Great Basin," in *History and Humanities,* ed. Francis X. Hartigan (Reno: University of Nevada Press, 1989), 105–20.

2. Richard Maxwell Brown, *Strain of Violence, Historical Studies of American Violence and Vigilantism* (Oxford: Oxford University Press, 1975), 104.

3. Terence Ranger and Paul Slack, eds., *Epidemics and Ideas: Essays on the Historical Perception of Pestilence* (Cambridge: Cambridge University Press, 1992); Catherine Gallagher and Thomas Laqueur, eds., *The Making of the Modern Body* (Berkeley: University of California Press, 1987); Charles E. Rosenberg and Janet Golden, eds., *Framing Disease: Studies in Cultural History* (New Brunswick, N.J.: Rutgers University Press, 1992).

4. From David Arnold, "Cholera and Colonialism," *Past and Present* 113 (1986): 118–51, quoted in Ranger and Slack, *Epidemics and Ideas,* 10.

5. Thomas McKeown, *The Origins of Human Disease* (Oxford: Blackwell, 1988).

6. The use of the term *framing* follows Rosenberg and Golden, *Framing Disease.*

7. On the emotional as well as conceptual features of scientific thought collectives, see Lorraine Daston, "The Moral Economy of Science," *Osiris* 10 (1995): 3–24; also Ludwik Fleck, *Genesis and Development of a Scientific Fact* [1935], ed. Thaddeus Trenn and Robert K. Merton, trans. Fred Bradley and Thaddeus Trenn (Chicago: University of Chicago Press, 1979).

8. Several oral histories include *Noah Smernoff, M.D.: A Nevada Physician* (1990), *Leslie Moren, M.D.: Fifty Years an Elko Doctor* (1992), and Anita Ernst Watson, *Reflections, Recollection, and Change: The Nevada State Board of Medical Examiners* (1996), all published by the University of Nevada, Reno, Oral History Program, R. T. King, director. Another promising project related to the region is Conevery Bolton, " 'The Health of the Country': Wellness, Sickness, and Sense of Place in the American West, 1803–1860" (Ph.D. diss. in progress, Harvard University).

1. The Significance of Regions in American Medical History

I am indebted to Sarah Pfatteicher and Jennifer Munger for their assistance in the preparation of this essay.

1. Ray Allen Billington, *Frederick Jackson Turner: Historian, Scholar, Teacher* (New York: Oxford University Press, 1973), 104–6, 181, 213–14. See also Frederick Jackson Turner's collection of essays, *The Significance of Sections in American History* (New York: Henry Holt, 1932).

2. Billington, *Frederick Jackson Turner*, 471; David R. Goldfield, "The New Regionalism," *Journal of Urban History* 10 (1984): 171–86; Richard Maxwell Brown, "The New Regionalism in America, 1970–1981," in *Regionalism and the Pacific Northwest*, ed. William G. Robbins, Robert J. Frank, and Richard E. Ross (Corvallis: Oregon State University Press, 1983), 37–96; Raymond D. Gastil, *Cultural Regions of the United States* (Seattle: University of Washington Press, 1975), 26–28, 226–46. See also Merrill Jensen, ed., *Regionalism in America* (Madison: University of Wisconsin Press, 1951); Frederick C. Luebke, "Regionalism and the Great Plains: Problems of Concept and Method," *Western Historical Quarterly* 15 (1984): 19–38; and D. W. Meinig, "The Continuous Shaping of America: A Prospectus for Geographers and Historians," *American Historical Review* 83 (1978): 1186–1205. For a useful bibliography, see Michael Steiner and Clarence Mondale, *Region and Regionalism in the United States: A Source Book for the Humanities and Social Sciences* (New York: Garland, 1988).

3. Fernand Braudel, *The Mediterranean and the Mediterranean World in the Age of Philip II*, 2 vols., trans. Sian Reynolds (New York: Harper & Row, 1972–73); Goldfield, "The New Regionalism," 174–77.

4. John Higham, "Multiculturalism and Universalism: A History and Critique," *American Quarterly* 45 (1993): 195–219, quotation on 202.

5. Charles Reagan Wilson and William Ferris, eds., *Encyclopedia of Southern Culture* (Chapel Hill: University of North Carolina Press, 1989); Carl Abbott, "Tracing the Trends in U.S. Regional History," *AHA Perspectives* (February 1990): 4–8.

6. Madge E. Pickard and R. Carlyle Buley, *The Midwest Pioneer: His Ills, Cures and Doctors* (New York: Henry Schuman, 1946), quotation on 199. These comments are based in part on the introduction to *Wisconsin Medicine: Historical Essays,* ed. Ronald L. Numbers and Judith Walzer Leavitt (Madison: University of Wisconsin Press, 1981), 3–11. Hippocrates, "On Airs, Waters, and Places," appears in *The Genuine Works of Hippocrates,* trans. Francis Adams (Baltimore: Williams & Wilkins, 1939), 19–42.

7. John Harley Warner, *The Therapeutic Perspective: Medical Practice, Knowledge, and Identity in America, 1820–1885* (Cambridge: Harvard University Press, 1986), quotation on 3.

8. Ibid., 69; John Harley Warner, "A Southern Medical Reform: The Meaning of the Antebellum Argument for Southern Medical Education," in *Science and Medicine in the Old South,* ed. Ronald L. Numbers and Todd L. Savitt (Baton Rouge: Louisiana State University Press, 1989), 179–205. James H. Cassedy, *Medicine and American Growth, 1800–1860* (Madison: University of Wisconsin Press, 1986), also explores antebellum regional rhetoric but dismisses it as "shallow sophistry" (81).

9. Warner, *Therapeutic Perspective*, 71.

10. Daniel Drake, *A Systematic Treatise, Historical, Etiological, and Practical, on the Principal Diseases of the Interior Valley of North America* (Cincinnati: Winthrop B. Smith,

1850), 1–5. Drake's *Second Series* was published in Philadelphia in 1854 by Lippincott, Grambo & Company.

11. Erwin H. Ackerknecht, "Diseases of the Middle West," in *Essays in the History of Medicine* (Chicago: Davis Lecture Committee, 1965), 168–81, quotation on 168. Ackerknecht acknowledged borrowing the saying from the French medical historian Charles Daremberg.

12. Drake, *Systematic Treatise* (1850), 2; James O. Breeden, "Disease as a Factor in Southern Distinctiveness," in *Disease and Distinctiveness in the American South,* ed. Todd L. Savitt and James Harvey Young (Knoxville: University of Tennessee Press, 1988), 1–28, quotation (from George Brown Tindall) on 12; John Ettling, *The Germ of Laziness: Rockefeller Philanthropy and Public Health in the New South* (Cambridge: Harvard University Press, 1981), 1.

13. K. David Patterson, "Disease Environments of the Antebellum South," in *Science and Medicine in the Old South,* ed. Numbers and Savitt, 152–65.

14. Elizabeth W. Etheridge, *The Butterfly Cast: A Social History of Pellagra in the South* (Westport, Conn.: Greenwood, 1972); Ettling, *Germ of Laziness;* Margaret Humphreys, *Yellow Fever and the South* (New Brunswick, N.J.: Rutgers University Press, 1992); John H. Ellis, *Yellow Fever & Public Health in the New South* (Lexington: University Press of Kentucky, 1992). See also the essays in *Disease and Distinctiveness in the American South,* ed. Savitt and Young; and *Science and Medicine in the Old South,* ed. Numbers and Savitt.

15. Erwin H. Ackerknecht, *Malaria in the Upper Mississippi* (Baltimore: Johns Hopkins Press, 1945); Victoria A. Harden, *Rocky Mountain Spotted Fever: History of a Twentieth-Century Disease* (Baltimore: Johns Hopkins University Press, 1990). For the Midwest, see also Peter T. Harstad, "Health in the Upper Mississippi River Valley, 1820 to 1861" (Ph.D. diss., University of Wisconsin, 1963).

16. Jake W. Spidle Jr., *Doctors of Medicine in New Mexico: A History of Health and Medical Practice, 1886–1986* (Albuquerque: University of New Mexico Press, 1986), 87–170, quotation on 91. See also Billy M. Jones, *Health-Seekers in the Southwest, 1817–1900* (Norman: University of Oklahoma Press, 1967).

17. *Roughing It* [1872], in *The Works of Mark Twain* (Berkeley: University of California Press, 1972), 164–65.

18. Frank B. Rogers, "The Rise and Decline of the Altitude Therapy of Tuberculosis," *Bulletin of the History of Medicine* 43 (1969): 1–16; Spidle, *Doctors of Medicine in New Mexico,* 87; Jones, *Health-Seekers in the Southwest,* 93, 121. On Colorado, see also Roy R. Anderson and Maxine Beaton, "From Pest Houses to Hospitals," in *A Century of Colorado Medicine, 1871–1971,* ed. Harvey T. Sethman (Denver: Colorado Medical Society, 1971), 33–37.

19. Spidle, *Doctors of Medicine in New Mexico,* 94, 163; Rogers, "Rise and Decline of Altitude Therapy," 15.

20. Rogers, "Rise and Decline of Altitude Therapy," 13; Jones, *Health-Seekers in the Southwest,* 190.

21. Abraham Flexner, *Medical Education in the United States and Canada* (New York: Carnegie Foundation for the Advancement of Teaching, 1910), 146, 151.

22. Ibid., 149–50, 197–99, 313. See also Richard W. Whithead and Robert L. Perkin, "Medical Education in Colorado, 1881–1971," in *A Century of Colorado Medicine,* ed. Sethman, 135–80.

23. Flexner, *Medical Education in the United States and Canada,* 150, 199.

24. Abraham Flexner, *An Autobiography* (New York: Simon & Schuster, 1960), 186–90. On regional rivalries in Wisconsin, see Ronald L. Numbers, "A Note on Medical Education in Wisconsin," in *Wisconsin Medicine,* ed. Numbers and Leavitt, 183.

25. James M. Faulkner, *Opportunity for Medical Education in Idaho/Montana/Nevada/Wyoming* (Boulder: Western Interstate Commission for Higher Education, 1964), vii, 5, 52; David C. Dale, "A Brief History of Graduate Medical Education in Washington, Alaska, Montana, and Idaho," *Western Journal of Medicine* 150 (1989): 476–77; Nancy M. Rockafellar and James W. Haviland, eds., *Saddlebags to Scanners: The First 100 Years of Medicine in Washington State* (Seattle: Washington State Medical Association, 1989), 192.

26. Daniel M. Fox, *Health Policies, Health Politics: The British and American Experience, 1911–1965* (Princeton: Princeton University Press, 1986), 16, 49.

27. Bess Furman, *A Profile of the United States Public Health Service, 1798–1948* (Washington, D.C.: Government Printing Office, n.d.), 350; Fitzhugh Mullan, *Plagues and Politics: The Story of the United States Health Service* (New York: Basic Books, 1989), 153; *The Wisconsin Regional Medical Program* (Milwaukee: n.p., [1969]), unpaginated brochure. During World War I the Public Health Service had created fourteen administrative regions; see Furman, *Profile,* 316.

28. Victor R. Fuchs, *Who Shall Live? Health, Economics, and Social Choice* (New York: Basic Books, 1974), 52–54; D. W. Meinig, "The Mormon Culture Region: Strategies and Patterns in the Geography of the American West, 1847–1964," *Annals of the Association of American Geographers* 55 (1965): 191–220, quotation on 191. On medicine in the Mormon culture region, see also Ralph T. Richards, *Of Medicine, Hospitals, and Doctors* (Salt Lake City: University of Utah Press, 1953); Claire Noall, *Guardians of the Hearth: Utah's Pioner Midwives and Women Doctors* (Bountiful, Utah: Horizon Publishers, 1974); Robert T. Divett, *Medicine and the Mormons: An Introduction to the History of Latter-Day Saint Health Care* (Bountiful, Utah: Horizon Publishers), 1981; and Lester E. Bush Jr., *Health and Medicine among the Latter-Day Saints: Science, Sense, and Scripture* (New York: Crossroad, 1993). On Nevada, see Edna B. Patterson, *Sagebrush Doctors* (Springfield, Utah: Art City Publishing, 1972), which includes a chapter on prostitution and public health.

29. Barron B. Beshoar, *Hippocrates in a Red Vest: The Biography of a Frontier Doctor* (Palo Alto, Calif.: American West, 1973), 155, 195; George N. Curtis, "Greetings from Utah," *Rocky Mountain Medical Journal* 35 (1938): 15–17. M. J. Smith, "The Rocky Mountain Medical Association and New Mexico Territorial Society," *New Mexico Medical Society Newsletter* 24 (January 1981): 2, which is based entirely on Beshoar's book, erroneously claims that the society was founded in 1881. I thank Tim Greer of the University of New Mexico Medical Center Library for supplying me with a copy of this article.

30. "Rocky Mountain Medical Journal (R.I.P.: 1938–79)," *Rocky Mountain Medical Journal* 76 (1979): 279–81; Curtis, "Greetings from Utah," 16; "A Voice for Medicine in the West," *Western Journal of Medicine* 120 (1974): 67.

31. "Salutatory," *Pacific Medical Record* 1 (January 1893): 11; "Local Medical Journals," ibid., 11–12. I am indebted to Phyllis A. Kauffman of the University of Wisconsin Middleton Health Sciences Library for making copies of the *Pacific Medical Record* and *Medical Sentinel* available to me. On the *Medical Sentinel,* see also O. Larsell, *The Doctor in Oregon: A Medical History* (Portland: Oregon Historical Society, 1947), 406–8.

32. See, e.g., Dale C. Smith, "Modern Surgery and the Development of Group Practice in the Midwest," *Caduceus* 2 (Autumn 1986): 1–39; and Paul C. Phillips, *Medicine in the Making of Montana* (Missoula: Montana State University Press, 1962), 34–40 on Jesuit missionaries as doctors.

2. Steaming Saints: Mormons and the Thomsonian Movement in Nineteenth-Century America

1. Unless otherwise noted, my source for Thomson's life and medical practice is his autobiography: *A Narrative of the Life and Medical Discoveries of Samuel Thomson,* 10th ed. (Columbus: Jarvis Pike & Company, 1833).

2. Samuel Thomson, *A New Guide to Health; or Botanic Family Physician,* 3d ed. (Boston: J. Q. Adams, 1835), 44.

3. *Thomsonian Recorder* 2 (1833): 96.

4. A number of secondary sources discuss the development of the Thomsonian movement as traced in this and the following paragraph. Chief among them are the works of Alex Berman: "The Thomsonian Movement and Its Relation to American Pharmacy and Medicine," *Bulletin of the History of Medicine* 25 (1951): 405–28, 519–38; "The Impact of the Nineteenth-Century Botanico-Medical Movement on American Pharmacy and Medicine" (Ph.D. diss., University of Wisconsin-Madison, 1954); and "Social Roots of the 19th Century Botanico-Medical Movement in the United States," *Actes VIIIe Congrès International d Histoire des Sciences* (1956): 561–65. Also quite useful is Joseph Kett, *The Formation of the American Medical Profession: The Role of Institutions, 1780–1860* (New Haven: Yale University Press, 1968), chap. 4: "Samuel Thomson and the Rise of Sectarian Medicine." Works of more limited value are William G. Rothstein, "The Botanical Movements and Orthodox Medicine," in *Other Healers: Unorthodox Medicine in America,* ed. Norman Gevitz (Baltimore: Johns Hopkins University Press, 1988); Madge E. Pickard and R. Carlyle Buley, *The Midwest Pioneer: His Ills, Cures, and Doctors* (New York: Henry Schuman, 1946), chap. 4: "The People's Doctors"; James O. Breeden, "Thomsonianism in Virginia," *Virginia Magazine of History and Biography* 82 (1974): 150–80; Frederick C. Waite, "Thomsonianism in Ohio," *Ohio State Archaeological and Historical Quarterly* 49 (1940): 322–31; James Harvey Young, *The Toadstool Millionaires: A Social History of Patent Medicines in America before Federal Regulation* (Princeton: Princeton University Press, 1961), chap. 4: "The Old Wizard"; and Daniel J. Wallace, "Thomsonians: The People's Doctors," *Clio Medica* 14 (1980): 169–86.

5. I explore this aspect of Thomsonianism more fully in "Every Woman a Physician: Women and Thomsonianism in Early Nineteenth-Century America" (MS).

6. Charles Rosenberg, *The Cholera Years: The United States in 1832, 1849, and 1866* (Chicago: University of Chicago Press, 1962), 162.

7. The database was compiled by searching Thomsonian journals for the names and other personal information on letter-to-the-editor writers and subscribers, local Friendly Botanic Society membership lists, etc.

8. While it is impossible to know the actual membership figures for all of these denominations, Edwin Scott Gaustad has done the next best thing and compiled the number of churches, which should be a fairly reliable indicator of overall membership strength. My percentages are calculated from the figures in his *Historical Atlas of Religion in America*, rev. ed. (New York: Harper & Row, 1976), 4, figs. 5 and 6.

9. There are a number of secondary sources for the early history of the LDS church. I have relied primarily on two: Douglas F. Tobler and Nelson B. Wadsworth, *The History of the Mormons in Photographs and Text: 1830 to the Present* (New York: St. Martin's Press, 1989); and Leonard J. Arrington and Davis Bitton, *The Mormon Experience: A History of the Latter-Day Saints* (New York: Alfred A. Knopf, 1979).

10. There is a fairly large body of historical writing on Mormon medicine and health care. Among the most useful are the works of Lester E. Bush Jr.: "The Mormon Tradition," in *Caring and Curing: Health and Medicine in the Western Religious Traditions,* ed. Ronald L. Numbers and Darrel W. Amundsen (New York: Macmillan, 1986), 397–420; and "The Word of Wisdom in Early Nineteenth-Century Perspective," *Dialogue: A Journal of Mormon Thought* 14 (Autumn 1981): 47–65. It is the latter work that notes the similarity between Mormon dietary prescriptions and contemporaneous health reform advocates. *Dialogue* devoted its fall 1979 issue to Mormon medicine and health care and included a number of historical essays. An overview worth mentioning is Robert T. Divett's *Medicine and the Mormons: An Introduction to the History of Latter-Day Saint Health Care* (Bountiful, Utah: Horizon Publishers, 1981). Less scholarly but of interest for the theme of this paper is John Heinerman, *Joseph Smith and Herbal Medicine,* 3d ed. (Monrovia, Calif.: Majority of One Press, 1980).

11. Divett, *Medicine and the Mormons,* chap. 2: "Health and the Smith Family," 21–37.

12. In addition to Divett's discussion of Williams in *Medicine and the Mormons,* 46–47, 84, see the biographical essay by his descendant, Frederick G. Williams, "Frederick Granger Williams of the First Presidency of the Church," *Brigham Young University Studies* 12 (1979): 243–61.

13. I explore the relationship between Thomsonianism and Methodism more fully in "The Wesleyan-Thomsonian 'Connection': Religious and Medical Dissent in the Early Republic" (MS, Department of the History of Science, University of Wisconsin-Madison, 1988).

14. Quinn's study is cited in Arrington and Bitton, *The Mormon Experience,* 29. The complete list is as follows: 10 Methodists, 5 Disciples of Christ, 3 Congregationalists, 2 Presbyterians, 1 Baptist, 1 Shaker, 8 unchurched, 4 unknown (several had more than one prior church).

15. Divett, *Medicine and the Mormons,* 92–97; Helen Richards Gardner, comp., *Levi Richards, 1799–1876: Some of His Ancestors and Descendants* (Logan, Utah: Unique Printing, 1973), 111–17.

16. Divett, *Medicine and the Mormons,* 92–97; Brigham Young, "The History of Willard Richards," *Millennial Star* 27 (1865): 118–20, 133–36, 150–52, 165–67.

17. Divett, *Medicine and the Mormons,* 84–88; Phyllis Richardson, "Thomsonian Influences in Early Mormon Utah History" (MS, LDS church History Division, Salt Lake City); Christine Croft Waters, "Pioneering Physicians in Utah" (master's thesis, University of Utah, 1976), 5.

18. Doctrine and Covenants, section 42 (cited in Bush, "The Mormon Tradition," 403).

19. Donald Q. Cannon and Lyndon W. Cook, eds., *The Far West Record: Minutes of the Church of Jesus Christ of Latter-Day Saints* (Salt Lake City: Deseret, 1983), 96–97.

20. Bush, "The Mormon Tradition," 404; Divett, *Medicine and the Mormons,* 152.

21. Chapter 32, title IX, "Offenses against Public Health," in *Acts, Resolutions and Memorials, Passed at the Several Annual Sessions, of the Legislative Assembly of the Territory of Utah, from 1851 to 1870 Inclusive* (Salt Lake City: Joseph, 1870), 59–60 (cited in Bush, "The Mormon Tradition," 407).

22. Richardson, "Thomsonian Influences in Early Mormon History," 12–13; Priddy Meeks, "Journal of Priddy Meeks," *Utah Historical Quarterly* 10 (1942): 163 (cited in Divett, *Medicine and the Mormons,* 115).

23. Ralph T. Richards, "The History of Medicine in Utah," *Bulletin of the University of Utah* 36 (1946): 8.

24. The professional Thomsonians in the East, although continuing to use the therapeutics as the basis of their practice, dropped "Thomsonian" from their self-description, adopting "botanico-medical" or "physio-medical" instead.

25. Austin Fife, "Pioneer Mormon Remedies," *Western Folklore* 16 (1957): 153–62.

26. Conrad Tarleton, letter to the editor, "The Great Pharmaceutical Cathalicon," *Southern Medical Reformer* 1 (1845): 155–56.

27. Meeks, "Journal of Priddy Meeks," 199–200 (cited in Heinerman, *Joseph Smith and Herbal Medicine,* 8–9).

3. Suicide in the Nevada Hinterlands: A Cultural Perspective

1. John L. McIntosh, *U.S.A. Suicide: 1991 Official Final Data,* Fact Sheet prepared for the American Association of Suicidology, 1993 (2459 S. Ash, Denver, CO 80222).

2. Sally S. Zanjani, "To Die in Goldfield: Mortality in the Last Boomtown on the Mining Frontier," *Western Historical Quarterly* 21 (1990): 47–69; also comments on "Suicide in the Nevada Hinterland: A Cultural Perspective" (paper presented at the symposium "Place and Practice: Regional Medicine, Health and Health Care in the Intermountain West," University of Nevada, Reno, October 1993).

3. Zanjani, "To Die in Goldfield," 1.

4. *Nevada Statistical Abstract, 1992* (Nevada Department of Administration, Carson City).

5. Maria Kilbourne, "Suicide, Meaning and Process" (Ph.D. diss., State University of New York at Albany, 1983).

6. Earl A. Grollman, *Suicide: Prevention, Intervention and Postvention* (Boston: Beacon Press, 1971), 59.

7. Comment made by the mother of my research assistant.

8. P. M. Meehan, P. W. O'Carrol, and J. Q. Jarvis, "Suicide in Nevada" (paper presented at 118th Annual Meeting of the American Public Health Association, September 30–October 4, 1990, New York).

9. *Nevada Statistical Abstract, 1994.*

10. Meehan et al., "Suicide in Nevada."

11. Norman Farberow, ed., *Suicide in Different Cultures* (Baltimore: University Park Press, 1975), xi–xviii.

12. Meehan et al., "Suicide in Nevada."

13. *Nevada Vital Statistics Report, 1989.*

14. *Reno Gazette Journal,* August 18, 1992.

15. *Nevada Vital Statistics Report, 1989.*

16. Ibid.

17. Jean Baechler, *Suicides,* trans. Barry Cooper (New York: Basic Books, 1979).

18. Coroner's records, White Pine County, Nevada, used with permission of White Pine County Sheriff's Office, Ely, Nevada.

19. Ibid.

20. Ibid.

21. Ibid.

22. Farberow, *Suicide in Different Cultures,* xiv–xv.

23. Kathleen Ann Long and Clarann Weinert, "Rural Nursing: Developing the Theory Base," *Scholarly Inquiry for Nursing Practice: An International Journal* 3 (1989): 123–26.

24. Coroner's records, White Pine County, Nevada.

25. Dayton Duncan, *Miles from Nowhere: Tales from America's Contemporary Frontier* (New York: Viking Penguin Books, 1983), 70–71.

26. Duncan, *Miles from Nowhere,* 146.

27. David Reynolds, Richard Kalish, and Norman Farberow, " A Cross-Ethnic Study of Suicide Attitudes and Expectations in the United States," in *Suicide in Different Cultures,* ed. Farberow, 35–50.

28. Ibid., 44.

29. John P. Webb and William Willard, "Six American Indian Patterns of Suicide," in *Suicide in Different Cultures,* ed. Farberow, 17–33.

30. Zanjani, "To Die in Goldfield."

31. Raymond Firth, "Suicide and Risk-Taking," in *Tikopia Ritual and Belief,* ed. Firth (London: Allen & Unwin, 1967), 119.

32. Long and Weinert, "Rural Nursing."

4. White Father Medicine and the Blackfeet, 1855–1955:
Native American Health and the Department of the Interior

1. Virginia Ruth Allen, "Health and Medical Care of the Southern. Plains Indians, 1868–1892" (Ph.D. diss., Oklahoma State University, 1973); idem, "Agency Physicians to the Southern Plains Indians, 1868–1900," *Bulletin of the History of Medicine* 49 (1975): 318–30; Anthony Godfrey, "Congressional-Indian Politics: Senate Survey of Conditions among the Indians of the United States" (Ph.D. diss., University of Utah, 1985); Diane Putney, "Fighting the Scourge: American Indian Morbidity and Federal Policy, 1897–1928" (Ph.D. diss., Marquette University, 1980); Francis Paul Prucha, *The Great Father: The United States Government and the American Indians,* vol. 2 (Lincoln: University of Nebraska Press, 1984), 841–63; Todd Benson, "Race, Health, and Power: The Federal Government and American Indian Health, 1909–1955" (Ph.D. diss., Stanford University, 1994).

2. See, e.g., H. L. Rieder, "Tuberculosis among American Indians of the Contiguous United States," *Public Health Report* 104 (1989): 653–57; and John W. Verano and Douglas H. Ubelaker, eds., *Disease and Demography in the Americas* (Washington, D.C.: Smithsonian Institution Press, 1992); William Clark, House of Representatives Register of Debates, 20th Cong., 1st sess., 1828, 1558, quotation in Laurence F. Schmeckebier, *The Office of Indian Affairs: Its History, Activities and Organization* (Baltimore: Johns Hopkins University Press, 1927), 41; Black Elk, *Black Elk Speaks* [as told to John G. Neihardt] (1932; reprint, Lincoln: University of Nebraska Press, 1989), 9; Charles E. Drew to William Clinton, in *Annual Report of the Board of Indian Commissioners, 1869* (Washington, D.C.: Government Printing Office, 1870), 67–69, quotation on 69.

3. As recorded in 22d Cong., 1st sess., 1832, H. Doc. 215, 526–705 in *House Journal,* and S. Doc. 211, 230–69 in *Senate Journal;* Michael K. Trimble, "The 1832 Inoculation Program on the Missouri River," in *Disease and Demography in the Americas,* ed. Verano and Ubelaker, 257–64.

4. George W. Manypenny, *Our Indian Wards* (Cincinnati: Robert Clarke, 1880), xxii.

5. See, e.g., Brenda J. Child, "A Bitter Lesson: Native Americans and the Government School Experience, 1890–19" (Ph.D. diss., University of Iowa, 1993); *Annual Report of the Department of Interior, 1904* (Washington, D.C.: Government Printing Office, 1905), 33–38, quotations on 33, 36.

6. Alfred Vaughan to A. Robinson, St. Louis, August 17, 1859, and April 2, 1860, Office of Indian Affairs, Letters Received 1824–81, Blackfeet 1855–69 (microfilm publication M234, roll 30); Alfred Sully to Ely S. Parker, "For the Indians in Montana for the year ending June 31, 1871," August 26, 1869, Records of the Montana Superintendency of Indian Affairs, 1867–1873 (M833, roll 3); Parker to Sully, October 18, 1869, and Sully to ?, October 20, 1869 (M833, roll 1). The 1870 incident is analyzed in Manypenny, *Our Indian Wards,* 272–93. Unless otherwise noted, all letters and reports cited are from Record Group 75, National Archives, Washington, D.C.

7. On general conditions, see, e.g., John Ewers, *The Blackfeet: Raiders of the Northwestern Plains* (Norman: University of Oklahoma Press, 1958); "The Blackfeet Indians,"

Appleton's Journal, July 1877, 37–43, quotation on 37; Cyrus Beede to H. Price, August 21, 1883, Letters Received, 1881–1907, 16070; "Indian Tribes in Northern Montana, etc.," 58th Cong., 2d sess., 1904, S. Doc. 255, ser. 4592, 1–21, quotation on 9.

8. Ales Hrdlička, "Tuberculosis among Certain Indian Tribes," *Bureau of American Ethnology Bulletin* 42 (1909): 4; *Contagious and Infectious Diseases among the Indians,* 62d Cong., 3d sess., 1913, S. Doc. 1038, ser. 6365, 43, 70.

9. *Annual Report of the Commissioner of Indian Affairs, 1889,* 12–13; Elsie E. Newton, "Sanitation and Medical Attendance—Blackfeet Reservation, 1914," December 31, 1914, Blackfeet Records, file 710, folder 4556-1915 (all files from Blackfeet records are in the National Archives, Record Group 75); *Annual Report of the Commissioner of Indian Affairs, 1916,* in George M. Kober et al. (Committee of the National Tuberculosis Association), *Tuberculosis among the North American Indians* (Washington, D.C.: Government Printing Office, 1923), 83; form letter from Office of Indian Affairs, file 710, folder 16849-1917.

10. Eugene W. Hill, Clifton M. Rosin, and Leslie J. Stauffer to E. B. Linnen, January 7, 1916, L. F. Michael to Commissioner, June 30, 1916, file 730, folder 74403-1916; C. J. Dewey to Commissioner, July 6, 1916, file 710; folder 55066-16; and Rosin to Commissioner, January 21, 1916, file 734, folder 15203-1916.

11. Kober et al., *Tuberculosis among the North American Indians,* 48–67; Hugh L. Scott, *Annual Report of the Board of Indian Commissioners, 1924* (Washington, D.C.: Government Printing Office, 1925), 24.

12. Lewis Meriam, *The Problem of Indian Administration* (Baltimore: Johns Hopkins University Press, 1928); Herman F. Schrader to James G. Townsend, November 1, 1935, file 700, folder 60794-1935; "Life on the Blackfeet Reservation," *Tushkahomman,* September 3, 1935, 4; H. W. Main to Chamber of Commerce, November 1931, file 723, folder 44401-1931; Stuart I. Hazlett to Burton K. Wheeler, July 26, 1937, and C. L. Graves to John Collier and William Zimmerman, September 18, 1937, file 720, folder 52026-1937.

13. Roy Nash, memo to council, farm agents, Father Halligan and Father Malman, Rev. Wilcox, teachers, editor of the *Chief,* Indian Office, December 26, 1941, file 734, folder 00-1941; "Physicians Monthly Reports Domiciliary and Out Patients, Ariz-Mont, 1936–1937," file 775, box 2; Rosalie I. Peterson to Commissioner, August 26, 1940, file 771, folder 59155-1940; Sallie Jeffries to Commissioner, March 5, 1940, report on February 7–11 inspection visit, file 771, folder 16800-1940; Lucille Ahnawake Hasting, inspection report received November 4, 1943, file 720, folder 44045.

14. Warren T. Creviston, inspection report on visits March 11–13 and April 19–21, 1947, file 770, folder 28587-1947; M. M. Young and K. Frances Cleave, undated report on Blackfeet hospital, file 770, folder 22045-1948; M. V. Hargett to Fred T. Foard, received September 12, 1949, and Hargett to Commissioner, September 30, 1947, file 770, folder 22045-1948; letters from the public are in file 720, folder 50403-1941.

15. *Annual Report of the Department of the Interior, 1904* (Washington, D.C.: Government Printing Office, 1905), 36, 38; Schmeckebier, *The Office of Indian Affairs,* 229. Information about the early health bureaucracy is primarily from this work and from Ruth M. Raup, *The Indian Health Program, from 1800–1955* (photocopy, Division of Indian Health, Public Health Service, 1959).

16. William H. Taft, quotation in Kober et al., *Tuberculosis among the North American Indians*, 75; Fred C. Campbell to Commissioner, February 29, 1924, file 732, folder 17484-1924; Elinor Gregg, *The Indians and the Nurse* (Norman: University of Oklahoma Press, 1965), 77–78; Campbell to Commissioner, March 16, 1925, Gregg, "Report on the Blackfeet Reservation," received December 2, 1924, file 720, folder 87370-1924.

17. Meriam, *The Problem of Indian Administration*, 212; C. E. Yates to Fred Campbell, April 8, 1924, Campbell to Commissioner, February 29, 1924, file 732, folder 17484-1924; Walter B. Stevens to E. B. Meritt, September 3, 1924, file 732, folder 67915-1924; quotation in Meritt to Campbell, June 24, 1924, file 731, folder 46358-1924; L. D. Fricks, Public Health Service inspection report, October 30–31, 1927, file 730, folder 53526-1927; Campbell to Commissioner, June 18, 1925, file 721, folder 63247-1924; Benson, "Race, Health, and Power," 201.

18. Benson, "Race, Health, and Power," 226; C. J. Rhoads to Forrest R. Stone, August 11, 1930, file 734, folder 41630-1930; on Stanford, see file 734, folder 44775-1945; Blanch M. Fuller to Franklin D. Roosevelt, October 29, 1936, file 721, folder 9271-1931; Collier to Stone, July 31, 1933, file 700, folder 34345-1933; Charles Edward Nagel to Schrader, September 13, 1933, file 700, no folder number.

19. Stone to Commissioner, September 24, 1930, Rhoads to Stone, October 8, 1930, file 734, folder 50722-1930; Stone to Commissioner, November 17, 1934, file 700, folder 58486-1934; Schrader to J. G. Townsend, November 1, 1935, file 700, folder 60794-1935.

20. Code of Federal Regulations, title 25, paragraphs 85.4 and 85.12, [n.d.]; Schrader to Townsend, August 3, 1940, file 734, folder 54382-1940; E—— K—— to Herman Schrader, January 20, 1943, file 721, folder 00-1943; R—— W—— to Stone, received December 14, 1931, C. J. Rhoads to Stone, January 7, 1932, file 732, folder 70800-1931; Schrader to Washington office, received February 16, 1931, file 700, folder 9736-1931.

21. "Indian Health Is Improving, Official Says," *Tushkahomman*, June 25, 1936, 2; "Health Director Brands T.B. as 'Killer of Indian Race,'" *Tushkahomman*, October 22, 1935, 1; "Two Important People Talk over the Indian Health Problem," *Tushkahomman*, October 15, 1935.

22. W. F. Braasch, B. J. Branton, and A. J. Chesley, "Survey of Medical Care among the Upper Midwest Indians," *Journal of the American Medical Association* [hereafter JAMA] 139 (1949): 220–26, quotation on 220; Everett R. Rhoades et al., "The Indian Health Service Record of Achievement," *Public Health Reports* 102 (1987): 356–60; Fred T. Foard, "The Federal Government and American Indians' Health," JAMA 142 (1950): 328–31, quotation on 329–30.

23. "Synopsis of Qualifications and Duties of Agency Physicians," Kiowa-Comanche Doctors File, Indian Archives Division, Oklahoma Historical Society, Oklahoma City, as noted in Allen, "Agency Physicians to the Southern Plains Indians," 319.

24. J. Armitage, "Second Quarter Report, 1872," in "Summary of Issues," F. A. Walker to J. A. Viall, October 23, 1872, William Ensign to Walker, December 4, 1872, E. P. Smith to James Wright, April 14, 1873, Ensign to Commissioner, quarterly report, May 1, 1873, and Smith to George B. Wright, May 13, 1873 (M833, roll 1); Joseph A. Murphy to Commissioner, September 1, 1914, E. B. Merrit to Murphy, September 21, 1914, file 710, folder

96466-14; L. F. Michael, inspection report, June 30, 1916, file 730, folder 74403-1916; Emil Krulish, inspection report, November 4, 1926, Forrest Stone to Commissioner, November 18, 1926, file 730, folder 52508-1926.

25. M. A. Miller to Commissioner Hiram Price, October 7, 1884, and R. A. Allen to Commissioner D. C. Atkins, July 8, 1885, Office of Indian Affairs, Letters Received, 1881–1907, nos. 19934 and 16113, respectively.

26. Schmeckebier, *The Office of Indian Affairs*, 288; Horace G. Wilson to Commissioner, March 22, 1919, file 420, folder 26789-1919; Warren L. O'Hara to Commissioner, July 25, 1935, file 700, no folder number; Elinor D. Gregg to Forrest Stone, January 11, 1935, file 700, no folder number; L. L. Elliott to Commissioner, December 16, 1939, file 709, folder 81135-1939.

27. Horace G. Wilson to Commissioner, November 22, 1920, file 710, folder 88200-1920; Wilson to Office of Indian Affairs, March 5, 1920, E. B. Meritt to Wilson, March 6, 1920, file 731, folder 19544-1920; Emil Krulish, inspection report, November 4, 1926, Forrest Stone to Commissioner, November 18, 1926, file 730, folder 52508-1926; Stone to Commissioner, April 25, 1931, file 721, folder 28609.

28. L. W. White and Allace S. White, inspection report, June 10, 1917, file 710, folder 61496-1917; on construction, see file 721, folder 124717-13; C. L. Ellis to Commissioner, July 7, 1915, file 721, folder 68519-1915; E. B. Meritt to Thomas Ferris, June 29, 1917, file 721, folder 56578-1917; Stone to Commissioner, April 7, 1933, file 700, folder 16060-1933; Lynne A. Fullerton, undated inspection report, file 700, folder 61267-1935; C. J. Rhoads to Forrest R. Stone, November 26, 1932, file 721, folder 47326.

29. *Annual Report of the Commission on Indian Affairs, 1886*, xli; *Annual Report of the Commission on Indian Affairs, 1889*, 12; Theodore F. Crabbe to Chief of Branch of Health [Fred Foard], August 1, 1950, file 734, folder 16857-1950.

30. *Annual Report of the Department of the Interior, 1941* (Washington, D.C.: Government Printing Office, 1942), 431; Braasch et al., "Survey of Medical Care." Figures for in-hospital births vary with the source; see, e.g., Kenneth Crain, "U.S. Hospitals Bringing Health to Native Americans, Eskimos," *Hospital Management* 53 (1942): 66–68.

31. George F. Lull to William H. Harrison, Chairman, Subcommittee on Indian Affairs, House of Representatives, April 20, 1953, in JAMA 152 (1953): 169; Theodore Taylor, *American Indian Policy* (Mt. Airy, Md.: Lomond, 1983); Kober et al., *Tuberculosis among the North American Indians*, 44. See also Donald L. Fixico, *Termination and Relocation: Federal Indian Policy, 1945–1960* (Albuquerque: University of New Mexico Press, 1986).

32. Foard, "The Federal Government and the American Indians' Health."

33. Ibid.; "Indian Health Laid to Parsimony," *New York Times*, March 7, 1951, 31; Foard, "The Health of the American Indians," *American Journal of Public Health* 39 (1949): 1403–6.

34. Foard, "The Federal Government and American Indians' Health," 329–30; Stephen J. Kunitz, *Disease Change and the Role of Medicine: The Navajo Experience* (Berkeley: University of California Press, 1983); idem, *Disease and Social Diversity: The European Impact on the Health of Non-Europeans* (Cambridge: Oxford University Press, 1994).

35. Diane D. Edwards, "Crossing the Medicine Line: Health Care and the Blackfoot Confederacy in the United States and Canada" (Ph.D. diss. University of Wisconsin-Madison, in progress); Frederick H. Abbott, *The Administration of Indian Affairs in Canada: Report of an Investigation Made in 1914 under the Direction of the [U.S.] Board of Indian Commissioners* (Washington, D.C.: Government Printing Office, 1915); Hana Samek, *The Blackfoot Confederacy, 1880–1920: A Comparative Study of Canadian and U.S. Indian Policy* (Albuquerque: University of New Mexico Press, 1987). For comparative studies, see Kunitz, *Disease and Social Diversity.*

36. H. Norman Old, "Sanitation Problems of the American Indians," *American Journal of Public Health* 43 (1953): 210–15, quotation on 211; "Spread of TB Laid to a New Source," *New York Times,* May 28, 1952, 27; Oliver LaFarge, quotationd in *Great Documents in American Indian History,* ed. Wayne Moquin and Charles Van Doren (New York: Praeger, 1973), 276.

5. The Scientific Construction of New Diseases: Rocky Mountain Spotted Fever and AIDS as Comparative Case Studies

1. On the sociology of scientific research, see Bruno Latour and Steve Woolgar, *Laboratory Life: The Construction of Scientific Facts,* 2d ed. (Princeton: Princeton University Press, 1986); Karin D. Knorr-Cetina, *The Manufacture of Knowledge: An Essay on the Constructivist and Contextual Nature of Science* (New York: Pergamon, 1981); and Michael Lynch, *Art and Artefact in Laboratory Science: A Study of Shop Work and Shop "Talk" in a Research Laboratory* (London: Routledge & Kegan Paul, 1985). For an overview of work in the history of medicine, see John Harley Warner, "Science in Medicine," *Osiris,* 2d ser., 1 (1985): 37–58.

2. I am using the term *paradigm* to mean an intellectual framework that provides the basic assumptions within which individual facts may be discovered and concepts such as "disease" may be described and elaborated. See Thomas Kuhn, *The Structure of Scientific Revolutions* (Chicago: University of Chicago Press, 1970).

3. There is a large literature on the history of the germ theory. A good recent overview and bibliography is Lois N. Magner, *A History of Medicine* (New York: Marcel Dekker, 1992), 305–33.

4. For histories of immunology, see Arthur M. Silverstein, *A History of Immunology* (San Diego: Academic Press, 1989); Debra Jan Bibel, *Milestones in Immunology: A Historical Exploration* (Madison, Wisc.: Science Tech Publishers, 1988).

5. Victoria A. Harden, *Rocky Mountain Spotted Fever: History of a Twentieth-Century Disease* (Baltimore: Johns Hopkins University Press, 1990), 1–3, 227–32.

6. Ibid., 3–4.

7. W. C. Rucker, "Rocky Mountain Spotted Fever," *Public Health Reports* [hereafter PHR] 27 (1912): 1471.

8. Marshall W. Wood, "Spotted Fever as Reported from Idaho," in U.S. War Department, *Report of the Surgeon General of the Army to the Secretary of War, 1896* (Washington, D.C.: Government Printing Office, 1896), 60; Edward E. Maxey, "Some Obser-

vations on the So-called Spotted Fever of Idaho," *Medical Sentinel* 7 (October 1899): 433–38.

9. "Tick-borne Infections in Colorado," *Journal of the American Medical Association* [hereafter JAMA] 94 (1930): 1172 (abstract); J. M. Braden, "Some Observations on Four Cases of Spotted Fever Occurring in Colorado," *Colorado Medicine* 3 (1906): 213–19; "RMSF—Colorado—Early History to 1929," Notebooks of Ralph R. Parker, Research Records of the Rocky Mountain Laboratory, Records of the National Institutes of Health, Record Group 443, National Archives and Records Administration, Washington, D.C. [hereafter R. R. Parker Notebooks]; Frederick D. Stricker, "The Prevalence and Distribution of Rocky Mountain Spotted Fever in Oregon," in "Rocky Mountain Spotted Fever," *Montana State Board of Health Special Bulletin* 26 (1923): 18–20, quotation on 18; "RMSF—Oregon—Early History to 1925," R. R. Parker Notebooks.

10. Albert B. Tonkin, "Incidence of Rocky Mountain Spotted Fever in Wyoming," in "Rocky Mountain Spotted Fever," *Montana State Board of Health Special Bulletin* 26 (1923): 23–27; "RMSF—Wyoming—Early History to 1926," R. R. Parker Notebooks.

11. On Washington, see A. U. Simpson, "Rocky Mountain Tick Fever in the State of Washington," in "Rocky Mountain Spotted Fever," *Montana State Board of Health Special Bulletin* 26 (1923): 20–23. On California, see F. L. Kelly, "Rocky Mountain Spotted Fever: Its Prevalence and Distribution in Modoc and Lassen Counties, California: A Preliminary Report," *California State Journal of Medicine* 14 (1916): 407–9; idem, "Rocky Mountain Spotted Fever in California," PHR 31 (1916): 2753–54; J. G. Cumming, "Rocky Mountain Spotted Fever in California," *Journal of Infectious Diseases* 21 (1917): 509–14; "RMSF—California—Early History to 1929," R. R. Parker Notebooks. On Utah and Nevada, see A. A. Robinson, "Rocky Mountain Spotted Fever, with Report of a Case," *Medical Record* 74 (1908): 913–22; "RMSF—Utah—Early History to 1931" and "RMSF—Nevada—Early History to 1928," R. R. Parker Notebooks.

12. Lewis and Clark traversed the Bitterroot early in the nineteenth century but mentioned no disease. Since they had been specifically commissioned to note medical problems among the native peoples, it is not unreasonable to presume that they neither observed spotted fever nor heard of its occurrence. Further, the Salish and Nez Percé tribes, who regularly visited the Bitterroot, did not report a long-standing knowledge of a malady resembling spotted fever when questioned by early twentieth-century researchers. See Reuben G. Thwaites, ed., *The Journals of Lewis and Clark,* 8 vols. (New York, 1905; reprint, Arno Press, 1969), 3:52–57, 5:246; Samuel Lloyd Cappious, "History of the Bitter Root Valley to 1914" (master's thesis, University of Washington, 1939), 6–10; Phyllis Twogood, Henry Grant, and Lena Bell, "History of Lewis & Clark expedition in the Bitter Root Valley," in *Bitterroot Trails,* 2 vols., ed. Bitter Root Valley Historical Society (Darby, Mont.: Professional Impressions, 1982), 1:37–45; Paul C. Phillips, *Medicine in the Making of Montana* (Missoula: Montana State University Press, 1962), 20–31; report of the investigation by Louis B. Wilson and William M. Chowning, in Montana State Board of Health, *First Biennial Report of the Montana State Board of Health from Its Creation March 15, 1901 to November 30, 1902* (Helena, [1903]), 28.

13. Harden, *Rocky Mountain Spotted Fever,* 14–15. For a broad view of human-micro-

organism interactions, see William H. McNeill, *Plagues and Peoples* (Garden City, N.Y.: Doubleday, 1976).

14. These theories are reported in Maxey, "Some Observations on the So-called Spotted Fever of Idaho," 434; and in Wood, "Spotted Fever as Reported from Idaho," 61, 63.

15. Report of the investigation by Louis B. Wilson and William M. Chowning; J. O. Cobb, "The So-Called 'Spotted Fever' of the Rocky Mountains—A New Disease in the Bitter Root Valley, Mont.," PHR 17 (1902): 1869.

16. Victoria A. Harden, "Rocky Mountain Spotted Fever Research and the Development of the Insect Vector Theory, 1900–1930," *Bulletin of the History of Medicine* 59 (1985): 449–66.

17. Louis B. Wilson and William M. Chowning, "Studies in Pyroplasmosis Hominis: ('Spotted Fever' or 'Tick Fever' of the Rocky Mountains)," *Journal of Infectious Diseases* 1 (1904): 31–33; Montana State Board of Health, *First Biennial Report*, 26–27. The spelling of this putative organism was later corrected to *Piroplasmosis* to conform with accepted zoological nomenclature.

18. Charles Wardell Stiles, "A Zoological Investigation into the Cause, Transmission, and Source of Rocky Mountain 'Spotted Fever,'" *U.S. Hygienic Laboratory Bulletin* 20 (1905).

19. Howard Taylor Ricketts, "The Transmission of Rocky Mountain Spotted Fever by the Bite of the Wood Tick (*Dermacentor occidentalis*)," JAMA 47 (1906): 358.

20. Rennie W. Doane, *Insects and Disease: A Popular Account of the Way in Which Insects May Spread or Cause Some of Our Common Diseases* (New York: Henry Holt, 1910), 32. For his pioneering research, Ricketts was honored posthumously by having the organisms that cause Rocky Mountain spotted fever and typhus named rickettsiae in his honor. The agent of spotted fever is even called *Rickettsia rickettsii*.

21. Robert Koch, "Die Ätiologie der Tuberkulose," in *Gesammelte Werke von Robert Koch*, 2 vols., ed. J. Schwalbe (Leipzig: Georg Thieme, 1912), 1: 467–565. An English translation of this paper is in idem, *The Aetiology of Tuberculosis*, trans. Dr. and Mrs. Max Pinner (New York: National Tuberculosis Association, 1922). Koch's postulates are as follows:

1. An alien structure must be exhibited in all cases of the disease.
2. The structure must be shown to be a living organism and must be distinguishable from all other microorganisms.
3. The distribution of microorganisms must correlate with and explain the disease phenomena.
4. The microorganism must be cultivated outside the diseased animal and isolated from all disease products that could be causally significant.
5. The pure isolated microorganism must be inoculated into test animals, which must then display the same symptoms as the original diseased animal.

Points 1, 2, and 3 embody the necessity argument, or absence argument, that without the organism no disease results; points 4 and 5 embody the sufficiency argument, that this specific organism will always cause a specific disease. Koch knew that host factors made proof of the sufficiency argument almost impossible except under special circumstances. For a fuller discussion of these issues with respect to spotted fever, see Victoria A. Harden, "Koch's Postulates and the Etiology of Rickettsial Diseases," *Journal of the History of Medicine and Allied Sciences* 42 (July 1987): 277–95.

22. While studying anthrax and wound infections, Koch grew bacterial cultures in liquid medium; hence he could not isolate a single bacterium and from it grow a "pure culture." In his work on cholera, Koch could not identify a suitable experimental animal in which to reproduce the disease.

23. Howard Taylor Ricketts, "A Micro-organism Which Apparently Has a Specific Relationship to Rocky Mountain Spotted Fever: A Preliminary Report," JAMA 52 (1909): 379–80; Ricketts to Thomas D. Tuttle, March 17, 1909, folder 1, "Rocky Mountain Spotted Fever, 1908–1911," box 1, "General Correspondence," Montana State Board of Health Records, RG 28, Montana State Archives.

24. S. Burt Wolbach, "Studies on Rocky Mountain Spotted Fever," *Journal of Medical Research* 41 (1919): 1–197. The first overview of rickettsial diseases taking into account the biochemical and electron microscope findings about viruses is *Virus and Rickettsial Diseases, with Especial Consideration of Their Public Health Significance,* proceedings of a symposium held at the Harvard School of Public Health, June 12–June 17, 1939 (Cambridge: Harvard University Press, 1940).

25. For a fuller discussion of this controversy, see Harden, *Rocky Mountain Spotted Fever,* 72–100.

26. Report of Louis B. Wilson and William M. Chowning, in Montana State Board of Health, *First Biennial Report,* 27.

27. Stiles, "A Zoological Investigation into the Cause, Transmission, and Source of Rocky Mountain 'Spotted Fever,'" 7. See also John F. Anderson, "Spotted Fever (Tick Fever) of the Rocky Mountains: A New Disease," *U.S. Hygienic Laboratory Bulletin* 14 (1903).

28. Nathan Banks, "A Revision of the Ixodoidea, or Ticks, of the United States," *U.S. Department of Agriculture Bulletin* 15 (1908). The species name, *venustus,* means "lovely, charming, or beautiful."

29. "Opinion 78: Case of Dermacentor andersoni vs. Dermacentor venustus," in "Opinions Rendered by the International Commission on Zoological Nomenclature: Opinions 78 to 81," *Smithsonian Miscellaneous Collections* 73, no. 2 (1924): 1–14.

30. See, e.g., Montana State Board of Entomology, *First Biennial Report, 1913–1914* (Helena, 1915), 12, 28.

31. Gerald M. Oppenheimer, "In the Eye of the Storm: The Epidemiological Construction of AIDS," in *AIDS: The Burdens of History,* ed. Elizabeth Fee and Daniel M. Fox (Berkeley: University of California Press, 1988), 267–300.

32. There is a large literature on AIDS. The earliest popular journalistic study is Randy Shilts, *And the Band Played On: Politics, People, and the AIDS Epidemic* (New York: St. Martin's Press, 1987); the first overview presented as a scholarly monograph is Mirko Grmek, *History of AIDS: Emergence and Origin of a Modern Pandemic,* trans. Russel C.

Maulitz and Jacalyn Duffin (Princeton: Princeton University Press, 1990), originally published as *Histoire du sida: Début et origine d'une pandémie actuelle* (Paris: Éditions Payot, 1989). Two collections of scholarly studies on AIDS are *AIDS: The Burdens of History,* ed. Elizabeth Fee and Daniel M. Fox (Berkeley: University of California Press, 1988); and Elizabeth Fee and Daniel M. Fox, *AIDS: The Making of a Chronic Disease* (Berkeley: University of California Press, 1992). On the difficulty of viral transmission, see Victoria A. Harden and Dennis Rodrigues, interview with Barbara Baird, March 17, 1993, NIH Clinical Center, Bethesda, Md.

33. Giuseppe Pantaleo, Cecilia Graziosi, James F. Demarets, et al., "HIV Infection Is Active and Progressive in Lymphoid Tissue during the Clinically Latent Stage of Disease," *Nature* 362 (1993): 355–58.

34. Shilts, *And the Band Played On,* 11–33.

35. See the summary of the meeting describing the disease in these groups in Arthur S. Levine to Vincent T. DaVita Jr., "Update on the Epidemic of Acquired Immunodeficiency–Kaposi Sarcoma–Opportunistic Infection," July 2, 1982, memorandum in "Kaposi's Sarcoma, July 1982" file, Intramural Research 5-15, Office of the Director Central Files, National Institutes of Health.

36. For example, in April 1982, a National Cancer Institute [hereafter NCI] administrator stated to a congressional committee, "I welcome this opportunity to appear before you today to discuss the Kaposi's sarcoma/opportunistic infections/acquired immunodeficiency syndrome." By the end of July 1982, however, NCI memoranda referring to the agency's draft Request for Applications for the disease had reversed the name. See "Statement by Bruce A. Chabner, M.D., Acting Director, Division of Cancer Treatment, National Cancer Institute, Department of Health and Human Services, before the Subcommittee on Health and the Environment, Committee on Energy and Commerce, House of Representatives, 13 April 1982," typescript; and Head, Medicine Section, Clinical Investigations Branch [hereafter CIB], Division of Cancer Treatment [hereafter DCT], NCI, to Acting Director, DCT, through Chief, CIB, Cancer Therapy Evaluation Program [hereafter CTEP], DCT and through Acting Associate Director, CTEP, DCT, "Acquired Immunodeficiency Syndrome RFA (Request for Applications)," memorandum dated July 23, 1982, both in "Kaposi's Sarcoma, 1981–1982," DCT files, NCI, copies in NIH Historical Office.

37. Gary W. Shannon, Gerald F. Pyle, and Rashid L. Bashshur, *The Geography of AIDS: Origins and Course of an Epidemic* (New York: Guilford Press, 1991), 61. Because there have been no national surveys of HIV seropositivity, the incidence and prevalence of infection with the AIDS virus must be inferred from data about reported cases of AIDS.

38. Ibid., 115, figs. 6.1 and 6.2.

39. Ibid., 116–17, figs. 6.3, 6.4, 6.5, and 6.6.

40. See their charts showing the incidence of cases in cities and in "the rest of" particular states, which convey the actual situation more clearly in ibid., 120, fig. 6.7, and 122, fig. 6.9.

41. Albert R. Jonsen and Jeff Stryker, eds., *The Social Impact of AIDS in the United States* (Washington, D.C.: National Academy Press, 1993), 7.

42. "*Pneumocystis Pneumonia*—Los Angeles," *Morbidity and Mortality Weekly Report* 30 (1981): 250; "Kaposi's Sarcoma and *Pneumocystis Pneumonia* among Homosexual Men—New York and California," in ibid., 305–8.

43. See description of agents surveyed at a National Institute of Allergy and Infectious Diseases workshop in April 1983 in Victoria A. Harden and Dennis Rodrigues, interview with Richard G. Wyatt, National Institutes of Health, Bethesda, Md., March 28, 1990; Public Health Service, "Fiscal Year 1985 Justification of Appropriation Estimates for Committee on Appropriations," supplementary budget data (Moyer material), administrative document, National Institutes of Health, 15.

44. R. C. Gallo, "The First Human Retrovirus," *Scientific American* 255, no. 6 (1986): 88–98; Gallo, *Virus Hunting: AIDS, Cancer, and the Human Retrovirus: A Story of Scientific Discovery* (New York: Basic Books, 1991). The designation HTLV originally stood for "human T-cell leukemia virus" in reference to the cancer caused by the virus. Later the "L" was changed to mean "lymphotrophic" to indicate that members of this class of viruses have an affinity for T-lymphocytes, whether or not leukemia results from infection.

45. There are many accounts, from various points of view, of the discovery of the AIDS virus. Some of the major ones include Robert C. Gallo and Luc Montagnier, "The Chronology of AIDS Research," *Nature* 326 (1987): 435–36; Gallo, *Virus Hunting*, 127–204; and John Crewdson, "The Great AIDS Quest," *Chicago Tribune*, November 19, 1989, sec. 5.

46. Alfred S. Evans, "Does HIV Cause AIDS? An Historical Perspective," *Journal of AIDS* 2 (1989): 107–13; Victoria A. Harden, "Koch's Postulates and the Etiology of AIDS: An Historical Perspective," *History and Philosophy of the Life Sciences* 14 (1992): 245–65.

47. Peter H. Duesberg, "Retroviruses as Carcinogens and Pathogens: Expectations and Reality," *Cancer Research* 47 (1987): 1199–1220; Duesberg, "Does HIV Cause AIDS?" *Journal of AIDS* 2 (1989): 514–15; Robert S. Root-Bernstein, *Rethinking AIDS: The Tragic Cost of Premature Consensus* (New York: Free Press, 1993); idem, "Do We Know the Cause(s) of AIDS?" *Perspectives in Biology and Medicine* (1990): 480–500.

48. Series of short papers in Policy Forum, *Science* 421 (1988): 514–17: Peter Duesberg, "HIV Is Not the Cause of AIDS"; "Blattner and Colleagues Respond to Duesberg"; William Blattner, Robert C. Gallo, and Howard M. Temin, "HIV Causes AIDS"; "Duesberg's Response to Blattner and Colleagues." See also interviews conducted by Victoria A. Harden and Dennis Rodrigues with William A. Blattner, March 2, 1990; and Anthony S. Fauci, June 29, 1993, copies of which are in the NIH Historical Office.

49. Françoise Barré-Sinoussi, Jean-Claude Chermann, F. Rey, et al., "Isolation of a T-Lymphotropic Retrovirus from a Patient at Risk for Acquired Immune Deficiency Syndrome," *Science* 220 (1983): 868–71.

50. The U.S. HTLV-III virus was announced in a series of four papers, all in *Science* 224 (1984): M. Popovic, M. G. Sarngadharan, E. Read, and R. C. Gallo, "A Method for Detection, Isolation and Continuous Production of Cytopathic Retroviruses (HTLV-III) from Patients with AIDS and Pre-AIDS," 497–500; R. C. Gallo, S. Z. Salahuddin, M. Popovic, et al., "Frequent Detection and Isolation of Cytopathic Retroviruses (HTLV-

III) from Patients with AIDS and at Risk for AIDS," 500–3; J. Schüpbach, M. Popovic, R. V. Gilden, et al., "Serological Analysis of a Subgroup of Human T-Lymphotropic Retroviruses (HTLV-III) Associated with AIDS," 503–5; and M. G. Sarngadharan, M. Popovic, L. Bruch, et al., "Antibodies Reactive with Human T-Lymphocyte Retroviruses (HTLV-III) in the Serum of Patients with AIDS," 506–8.

51. Gallo and Montagnier, "The Chronology of AIDS Research," 435–36.

52. J. Coffin, A. Haase, J. A. Levy, et al., "What to Call the AIDS Virus?" *Nature* 321 (1986): 10; idem, "Human Immunodeficiency Viruses," *Science* 232 (1986): 697.

6. "Many Have Died and Others Must": The Silicosis Epidemic in Western Hardrock Mining, 1900–1925

1. Abram S. Benenson, ed., *Control of Communicable Diseases in Man,* 13th ed. (Washington, D.C.: American Public Health Association, 1981), 411; Judith S. Mausner and Anita K. Bahn, *Epidemiology: An Introductory Text* (Philadelphia: W. B. Saunders, 1974), 22; Brian MacMahon and Thomas F. Pugh, *Epidemiology: Principles and Methods* (Boston: Little, Brown, 1970), 1–4, quotation on 2; Gary D. Friedman, *Primer of Epidemiology,* 3d ed. (New York: McGraw-Hill, 1987), 78–80; cf. Charles E. Rosenberg, *Explaining Epidemics and Other Studies in the History of Medicine* (Cambridge: Cambridge University Press, 1992), 278–304. For a study that treats benzidine-induced cancer as an epidemic occupational disease, see David Michaels, "Waiting for the Body Count: Corporate Decision Making and Bladder Cancer in the U.S. Dye Industry," *Medical Anthropology Quarterly,* n.s., 2 (September 1988): 215–32.

2. Dan DeQuille, "Miners' Consumption," *Mining and Scientific Press,* February 18, 1893, 106; George Kislingbury to Editor, n.d., *Mining and Scientific Press,* February 8, 1890, 92; Otis E. Young Jr., *Black Powder and Hand Steel: Miners and Machines on the Old Western Frontier* (Norman: University of Oklahoma Press, 1975), 10; Mabel Barbee Lee, *Cripple Creek Days* (Garden City, N.Y.: Doubleday, 1958), *passim,* esp. 62–63, 129.

3. Editorial, *Engineering and Mining Journal,* June 2, 1904, 870; U.S. Bureau of the Census, *Special Reports: Mines and Quarries, 1902* (Washington, D.C.: Government Printing Office, 1905), 529–30, 477; Treve Holman, "Historical Relationship of Mining, Silicosis, and Rock Removal," *British Journal of Industrial Medicine* 4 (January 1947): 9–13; Young, *Black Powder,* 36; Mark Wyman, *Hardrock Epic: Western Miners and the Industrial Revolution, 1860–1910* (Berkeley: University of California Press, 1979), 84–117; *Silverton (Colo.) Weekly Miner,* January 13, 1905; Alice Hamilton, *Exploring the Dangerous Trades* (1943; reprint, Boston: Northeastern University Press, 1985), 217–22; Ross B. Moudy, "The Story of a Cripple Creek Miner," *Independent,* August 18, 1904, 380.

4. Guy Louis Rocha, "Regulating Public Health in Nevada: The Pioneering Efforts of Dr. Simeon Lemuel Lee," *Nevada Historical Society Quarterly* 29 (Fall 1986): 203; James H. Cassedy, "The Registration Area and American Vital Statistics: Development of a Health Research Resource, 1885–1915," *Bulletin of the History of Medicine* 39 (May–June 1965): 221–31, esp. 223, 225. Epidemiological data on silicosis remained inadequate, to say the least, for decades after the turn of the century. See H. N. Doyle et al., "Accomplish-

ments in the Epidemiologic Study of Silicosis in the United States," *Archives of Industrial Health* 12 (July 1955): 48–55, esp. 50: "Statistics on the incidence of occupational diseases, including silicosis, have always been notoriously poor in the United States."

5. John M. Townley, "The Delamar Boom: Development of a Small, One-Company Mining District in the Great Basin," *Nevada Historical Society Quarterly* 15 (Spring 1972): 3–9; James W. Hulce, *Lincoln County, Nevada: 1864–1909* (Reno: University of Nevada Press, 1971), 51–54; *Mining and Scientific Press,* June 29, 1895, 407; *DeLamar (Nev.) Lode,* April 19, 1898.

6. *DeLamar Lode,* April 1, 1895, September 7, 1896, May 22, 1900; *Mining and Scientific Press,* April 21, 1900, 435–36; *Engineering and Mining Journal,* December 14, 1918, 1038.

7. William W. Betts, "Chalicosis Pulmonum, or Chronic Interstitial Pneumonia Induced by Stone Dust," *Journal of the American Medical Association* 34 (January 13, 1900): 70; *DeLamar Lode,* June 13, 1899, April 15, 1895; *Salt Lake Tribune,* January 1, 1900, reprinted in *DeLamar Lode,* January 16, 1900.

8. John M. Peters, "Silicosis," in *Occupational Respiratory Diseases,* U.S. Department of Health and Human Services, National Institute for Occupational Safety and Health Publication 86-102 (Washington, D.C.: Government Printing Office, 1986), 219–37; Daniel E. Banks, "Acute Silicosis," in ibid., 239–41; Alan Derickson, *Workers' Health, Workers' Democracy: The Western Miners' Struggle, 1891–1925* (Ithaca: Cornell University Press, 1988), 45–49. On the changing natural history and clinical picture of silicosis in mining and several other industries, see David Rosner and Gerald Markowitz, *Deadly Dust: Silicosis and the Politics of Occupational Disease in Twentieth-Century America* (Princeton: Princeton University Press, 1991), *passim,* esp. 6–11.

9. Betts, "Chalicosis Pulmonum," 70–72, esp. 70; *Owyhee Avalanche* (Silver City, Ida.), September 8, 1899; *DeLamar Lode,* June 13, 1899. For an account of the most infamous outbreak of acute silicosis and the difficulties of ascertaining the death toll at an isolated work site (a water tunnel construction project in rural West Virginia), see Martin Cherniack, *The Hawk's Nest Incident: America's Worst Industrial Disaster* (New Haven: Yale University Press, 1986).

10. Betts, "Chalicosis Pulmonum," 70–74, esp. 71, 70; *DeLamar Lode,* September 5, October 3, 1899, April 30, 1901; *Tonopah (Nev.) Bonanza,* June 14, 1902. For a comparative perspective on this subject, see Alan Derickson, "Industrial Refugees: The Migration of Silicotics from the Mines of North America and South Africa in the Early Twentieth Century," *Labor History* 29 (Winter 1988): 66–89. For evidence that migration led to underrecognition of pneumoconiosis, see Sally S. Zanjani, "To Die in Goldfield: Mortality in the Last Boomtown on the Mining Frontier," *Western Historical Quarterly* 21 (February 1990): 58–59.

11. Alfred S. Warthin, "Silicosis," in *A Reference Handbook of the Medical Sciences,* vol. 7, ed. Albert H. Buck (New York: William Wood, 1904), 214; *San Miguel Examiner* (Telluride, Colo.), April 11, 1903, April 1, 1905; *Silverton Weekly Miner,* May 20, 1904, April 28, 1905, May 8, September 18, 1908; *Rhyolite (Nev.) Daily Bulletin,* January 12, 28, 1909; *Mining and Scientific Press,* October 8, 1910, 472, December 31, 1910, 859–60; cf. Robert H. Shikes, *Rocky Mountain Medicine: Doctors, Drugs, and Disease in Early Colorado* (Boulder: Johnson Books, 1986), 42.

12. John Vickers and John Driscoll testimony, January 30, 1911, in "Proceedings of the Joint Committee . . . to Investigate . . . Ventilation of the Mines," reprinted in U.S. Commission on Industrial Relations, *Final Report and Testimony*, 11 vols., 64th Cong., 1st sess., S. Doc. 415 (Washington, D.C.: Government Printing Office, 1916), 4:3925, 3939; Transvaal, *Report of the Miners' Phthisis Commission, 1902–1903* (Pretoria: Government Printing and Stationery Office, n.d.); Great Britain, *Report to the Secretary of State for the Home Department on the Health of Cornish Miners*, by J. S. Haldane, Joseph S. Martin, and R. Arthur Thomas, Cd. 2091 (London: His Majesty's Stationery Office, 1904); *Mining and Scientific Press*, December 17, 1910, 818.

13. Vernon H. Jensen, *Heritage of Conflict: Labor Relations in the Nonferrous Metals Industry up to 1930* (Ithaca: Cornell University Press, 1950); William D. Haywood, *Bill Haywood's Book: The Autobiography of William D. Haywood* (New York: International Publishers, 1929), 62ff.; Melvyn Dubofsky, "The Origins of Western Working Class Radicalism, 1890–1905," *Labor History* 7 (Spring 1966): 131–54; John R. Commons et al., *History of Labor in the United States, 1896–1932*, vol. 4: *Labor Movements*, by Selig Perlman and Philip Taft (New York: Macmillan, 1935), 169ff.; George G. Suggs Jr., *Colorado's War on Militant Unionism: James H. Peabody and the Western Federation of Miners* (Detroit: Wayne State University Press, 1972); James W. Byrkit, *Forging the Copper Collar: Arizona's Labor-Management War of 1901–1921* (Tucson: University of Arizona Press, 1982); Russell R. Elliott, *Radical Labor in the Nevada Mining Booms, 1900–1920* (Carson City: State Printing Office, 1963); Guy L. Rocha, "Radical Labor Struggles in the Tonopah-Goldfield Mining District, 1901–1922," *Nevada Historical Society Quarterly* 20 (Spring 1977): 3–45.

14. John C. Lowney to Editor, November 23, 1908, *Miners' Magazine* (Denver), December 10, 1908, 10–11; Lowney to Editor, March 16, 1909, *Miners' Magazine*, March 25, 1909, 11; Montana, *Laws, Resolutions and Memorials, 1911* (Helena: State Publishing Company, n.d.), 135–37.

15. Arizona, *Acts, Resolutions and Memorials, 1912, Regular Session* (Phoenix: McNeil, 1912), quotation on 105; Joseph D. Cannon, "What Has the Western Federation . . . Done," *Miners' Magazine*, August 17, 1916; J. Tom Lewis to Members of Organized Labor, n.d., *Arizona Labor Journal*, September 8, 1916, 2; Arizona, *Revised Statutes, 1913*, 2 vols. (Phoenix: McNeil, 1913), 1:1371; Derickson, *Workers' Health, Workers' Democracy*, 164–67.

16. For another rare instance of aggressive public policy to prevent occupational disease during this period, see R. Alton Lee, "The Eradication of Phossy Jaw: A Unique Development of Federal Police Power," *Historian* 29 (November 1966): 1–21; Jean Spencer Felton, "Phosphorus Necrosis—A Classical Occupational Disease," *American Journal of Industrial Medicine* 3 (1982): 77–120, esp. 95–104.

17. Nevada, Inspector of Mines, *Annual Report, 1912* (Carson City: State Printing Office, 1913), 9–11, Ryan quotations on 10 and 11; Western Federation of Miners, *Official Proceedings of the Twentieth Annual Convention, 1912* (Denver: Great Western, 1912), 190–91; Nevada, Board of Health, *Biennial Report, 1912* (Carson City: State Printing Office, 1913). On the early development of the Nevada Board of Health, see Rocha, "Regulating Public Health in Nevada," 201–9.

18. Executive Board, Western Federation of Miners, Minute Book, 3:96 (August 1,

1912), 115–16 (January 13, 1913), 127 (January 20, 1913), and opposite 131 (January 23, 1913), all in Western Federation of Miners–International Union of Mine, Mill and Smelter Workers Archives, Western Historical Collections, Norlin Library, University of Colorado, Boulder, vol. 3; *Miners' Magazine,* February 27, 1913, 10; Nevada, *Statutes, 1913* (Carson City: State Printing Office, 1913), 167–68, 305. For further discussion of the Nevada legislation and subsequent reforms in Idaho, British Columbia, and Ontario, see Derickson, *Workers' Health, Workers' Democracy,* 166–69. For an interpretation that purports to show the union's inaction, see James C. Foster, "Western Miners and Silicosis: 'The Scourge of the Underground Toiler,' 1890–1943," *Industrial and Labor Relations Review* 37 (April 1984): 371–85, esp. 371–72, 383–85.

19. Western Federation of Miners, *Official Proceedings of the Twenty-first Consecutive and First Biennial Convention, 1914* (Denver: Great Western, 1914), appendix, 37 (Moyer quotation), 82–83; Derickson, *Workers' Health, Workers' Democracy,* 180–82. For an account of the efforts to win compensation for silicosis in Arizona after 1925, albeit one that overlooks a decade of WFM agitation on this issue before the mid-1920s, see James C. Foster, *"The Western Dilemma:* Miners, Silicosis, and Compensation," *Labor History* 26 (Spring 1985): 278–82.

20. Doyle et al., "Accomplishments in Epidemiologic Study," 48–49. Analytical occupational epidemiology commenced in the 1920s with a federal investigation of granite workers in Vermont; see ibid., 49; A. E. Russell et al., *The Health of Workers in Dusty Trades: II. Exposure to Siliceous Dust (Granite Industry),* Public Health Bulletin 187 (Washington, D.C.: Government Printing Office, 1929).

21. S. C. Hotchkiss, "Occupational Diseases in the Mining Industry," *American Labor Legislation Review* 2 (February 1912): 131–39.

22. A. J. Lanza, *Miners' Consumption: A Study of 433 Cases of the Disease among Zinc Miners in Southwestern Missouri,* Public Health Bulletin 85 (Washington, D.C.: Government Printing Office, 1917), 14–26, 30; Edwin Higgins et al., *Siliceous Dust in Relation to Pulmonary Disease among Miners in the Joplin District,* U.S. Bureau of Mines Bulletin 132 (Washington, D.C.: Government Printing Office, 1917); Alan Derickson, "Federal Intervention in the Joplin Silicosis Epidemic, 1911–1916," *Bulletin of the History of Medicine* 62 (Summer 1988): 236–51.

23. Daniel Harrington to George S. Rice, June 26, 1916 (quotations), U.S. Bureau of Mines Records, RG 70, General Records, 1910–1950, box 237, file 54854.1, National Archives, Washington National Records Center, Suitland, Md. [hereafter NA]; A. J. Lanza and D. Harrington, "Preliminary Report of Investigation of Mountain View Mine, Butte, Montana, as to Hygienic Condition of Working Places," n.d. [ca. October 1916], *passim,* esp. 20–26, U.S. Public Health Service Records, RG 90, General Files, 1897–1923, box 500-L, file 5153, NA; Daniel Harrington, *Underground Ventilation at Butte,* U.S. Bureau of Mines Bulletin 204 (Washington, D.C.: Government Printing Office, 1923), *passim,* esp. 2; Daniel Harrington and A. J. Lanza, *Miners' Consumption in the Mines of Butte, Montana: Preliminary Report of an Investigation Made in the Years 1916–1919,* U.S. Bureau of Mines Technical Paper 260 (Washington, D.C.: Government Printing Office, 1921), 8–10.

24. Harrington and Lanza, *Miners' Consumption,* 5, 10–12; Van H. Manning to C. F. Kelley, March 10, 1917, U.S. Bureau of Mines Records, RG 70, General Records, 1910–1950, box 290, file 59203; G. S. Rice and R. R. Sayers, *Review of Safety and Health Conditions in the Mines at Butte,* U.S. Bureau of Mines Bulletin 257 (Washington, D.C.: Government Printing Office, 1925), ii.

25. U.S. Surgeon General, *Annual Report . . . for the Fiscal Year 1918* (Washington, D.C.: Government Printing Office, 1918), quotation on 45; *Engineering and Mining Journal,* May 24, 1919, 936; *Miners' Magazine,* May 1921, 7.

26. *Tonopah (Nev.) Mining Reporter,* December 10, 1921, 2 (quotation); *Tonopah Daily Bonanza,* December 15, 1921, 1; Cleve E. Kindall to R. R. Sayers, July 29, 1922, U.S. Bureau of Mines Records, RG 70, Records of the Office of the Chief Surgeon, 1916–1933, box 84, file 032.1; E. R. Sayres [*sic*—R. R. Sayers], E. R. Hayhurst, and A. J. Lanza, "Status of Silicosis," *American Journal of Public Health* 19 (June 1929): 636.

27. [Sayers] et al., "Status of Silicosis," 636; "Tom Reed Gold Mines Co. Supplementary Report," n.d. [1922], U.S. Bureau of Mines Records, RG 70, Records of the Office of the Chief Surgeon, 1916–1933, box 84, file 032.1; D. Harrington to E. D. Gardner, April 25, 1922, ibid., file 132.1; Harrington to B. O. Pickard, May 22, 1922, ibid.

28. Derickson, *Workers' Health, Workers' Democracy,* 50–52. Federal officials approached the issue but then backed away from making a prevalence estimate for the industry. See Rice and Sayers, *Review of Safety and Health Conditions in the Mines at Butte,* 14–15; R. R. Sayers, *Silicosis among Miners,* U.S. Bureau of Mines Technical Paper 372 (Washington, D.C.: Government Printing Office, 1925), 3–5.

29. On the control of silicosis, see W. O. Borcherdt, "Abatement of Dust from Drilling Operations by the Use of Water Drills," in *Proceedings of the National Safety Council Seventh Annual Safety Congress, 1918* (n.p., n.d.), 1034–42; *Engineering and Mining Journal-Press,* June 17, 1922, 1055; Charles A. Mitke, "Metal-Mine Ventilation in the Southwest," *Transactions of the American Institute of Mining and Metallurgical Engineers* 68 (1923): 377–86; D. Harrington, "Report of Committee on Metal Mine Ventilation," *Transactions of the American Institute of Mining and Metallurgical Engineers* 75 (1927): 141, 143; John W. Flinn and Robert S. Flinn, "Pneumonoconiosis," *Southwestern Medicine* 14 (July 1930): 329; Rice and Sayers, *Review of Safety and Health Conditions in the Mines at Butte,* iii–iv, 16–20, 27; Harrington, *Underground Ventilation at Butte, passim,* esp. iii; Derickson, *Workers' Health, Workers' Democracy,* 173. On the persistence of silicosis in western hardrock mining long after 1925, see Waldemar Dreessen et al., *Health and Working Environment of Nonferrous Metal Mine Workers,* Public Health Bulletin 277 (Washington, D.C.: Government Printing Office, 1942); Robert H. Flinn et al., *Silicosis in the Metal Mining Industry: A Revaluation, 1958–1961,* PHS Publication 1076, U.S. Public Health Service and U.S. Bureau of Mines (Washington, D.C.: Government Printing Office, 1963); Marcus M. Key and Howard E. Ayer, "Silicosis in Hard-Rock Mining," *Journal of Occupational Medicine* 14 (November 1972): 863–65; Rosner and Markowitz, *Deadly Dust,* 198–208. On pneumoconiosis in the tri-state district of Oklahoma, Missouri, and Kansas in the second quarter of the century, see Alan Derickson, " 'On the Dump Heap': Employee Medical Screening in the Tri-State Zinc-Lead Industry, 1924–

1932," *Business History Review* 62 (Winter 1988): 656–77; Rosner and Markowitz, *Deadly Dust*, 135–67.

7. Frontier Nursing: The Deaconess Experience in Montana, 1890–1960

1. Vern Bullough and Bonnie Bullough, *The Care of the Sick: The Emergence of Modern Nursing* (New York: Prodist, 1978), 236.

2. Norman Cousins, *Anatomy of an Illness as Perceived by the Patient: Reflections on Healing and Regeneration* (New York: Norton, 1979), 154.

3. Eduard Seidler, *Geschichte der Pflege des Kranken Menschen* (Stuttgart: Kohlhammer, 1977), 12.

4. Mabel E. Tuchserer, M.D., *Petticoat and Stethoscope: A Montana Legend,* ed. John A. Forssen (Missoula: Bitterroot Litho, 1978); Seidler, *Geschichte,* 69–85, 185–91; Leonard Brewer, *First 100 Years: Being a Review of the Beginnings, Growth and Development of the Montana Medical Association in Commemoration of the Centennial Year* (Missoula: Bitterroot Litho, 1978), esp. xiii–xvii, 1–15.

5. Sister Mary Carol Conroy, S.C.L., "The Historical Development of the Health Care Ministry of the Sisters of Charity of Leavenworth" (Ph.D. diss., Kansas State University, 1984); Sister Julia Gilmore, S.C.L., *Come North!* (New York: McMullen Books, 1951); Anne L. Austin, *History of Nursing Source Book* (New York: G. P. Putnam's Sons, 1957); Anna Pearl Sherrick, Jeannie M. Claus, and John P. Parker, *History of the Montana State University School of Nursing: A Story of Professional Development* (Bozeman: Big Sky Books, 1983); Anna Pearl Sherrick, Mary D. Munger, and Stanley R. Davison, *Nursing in Montana* (Great Falls: Tribune Printing, n.d. [1960?]); Bonnie Bullough, Vern L. Bullough, and Barrett Elcano, *Nursing: A Historical Bibliography* (New York: Garland, 1981).

The following list of Montana hospitals is correct up to 1960. Several had already closed by that date (e.g., St. John's in Helena, which was destroyed by an earthquake in 1935).

Catholic hospitals: St. Johns, Helena; St. Joseph's, Deer Lodge; St. Mary's, Virginia City; St. James, Butte; St. Ann's, Anaconda; St. Vincent, Billings; St. Patrick, Missoula; St. Clare, Fort Benton; Columbus, Great Falls; Kalispell General; St. Joseph's, Lewistown; Holy Rosary, Miles City; St. Joseph's, Polson; St. Mary's, Conrad; Sacred Hart, Havre.

Deaconess hospitals: Montana Deaconess, Great Falls; Frances Mahon, Glasgow; Bozeman Deaconess, Bozeman; Kennedy Deaconess, Havre; Community Memorial, Sidney; Billings Deaconess, Billings. In addition, there were industrial hospitals operated by Great Northern Railroad; two veterans' hospitals, one in Miles City, the other in Helena; several units of the state system; specialized children's units like Shodair, in Helena; Bureau of Indian Affairs and Indian Health Service facilities on the several reservations; joint philanthropic and state hospitals in Dillon and Hamilton; and in 1960 there were a total of thirty-six small hospitals scattered throughout the state.

6. Bullough and Bullough, *The Care of the Sick,* 75–103; Seidler, *Geschichte,* 191; Flieder said of nursing: "Schwierig ist solcher Beruf" (Difficult is the calling). On Flied-

ner, see *The Life of Pastor Fliedner of Kaiserwerth,* trans. from the German by Catherine Winkworth (New York: Longmans, Green, 1867).

7. Among her other talents Florence Nightingale was a gifted statistician. See Cecil Woodham-Smith, *Florence Nightingale 1820–1910* (New York: McGraw-Hill, 1951); Lytton Strachey, *Eminent Victorians* (New York: G. P. Putnam's Sons, 1918).

8. Marie Gallison, *The Ministry of Women: 100 Years of Women's Work at Kaiserwerth 1836–1936* (London: Lutterworth Press, 1926).

9. "The sleeping porches were in use the entire year, no matter how cold the weather was. There was considerable talking and laughing among ourselves at bedtime. The story was told of some people living nearby who were having company one evening. The guests inquired about where all the noise and laughter were taking place. The hostess told them, 'It is just the nurses going to bed' " (quoted in Ruth Strandness McCullough, "The Influence of the Nightingale Principles on Four Montana Deaconess Hospital Training Schools" [MS, December 1969, Montana State University, Bozeman], 139–44).

10. Christian Golder, *History of the Deaconess Movement in 1903* (Great Falls: n.p., n.d.); Sherrick et al., *History of Montana State University School of Nursing;* McCullough, "Nightingale Principles."

11. E. Augusta Ariss, *Historical Sketch of the Montana State Association of Registered Nurses and Related Organizations* (n.p., n.d. [probably 1937]).

12. Sherrick et al., *Nursing in Montana;* McCullough, "Nightingale Principles," 94ff.

13. The pledge is printed inside the front cover of Sherrick et al., *Nursing in Montana.* As befits the frontier, above the pledge is a photograph of the state capitol; below it a herd of bison.

14. Generally, established nurses like Miss Ariss and Miss Sherrick stressed the helpfulness of physicians; their literature, however, stressed that the nurses' professional "family" consisted of other nurses and alumni. There was little interaction across that gulf; see Sherrick et al., *Nursing in Montana;* McCullough, "Nightingale Principles," 141–45.

15. McCullough, "Nightingale Principles," 98–99.

16. Ibid., 100.

17. Ibid., 103.

18. Miss Ariss, Montana Methodist Conference Report (August 21, 1928), cited in McCullough, "Nightingale Principles," 106; Sherrick et al., *Nursing in Montana,* 55–66. The latter includes a table showing that in 1919 there were approximately 265 students enrolled in fifteen schools of nursing; in 1960 there were 617 students in four schools. Given the increase in collegiate populations both nationally and in Montana, that increase represents a net loss of interest in the field. Bullough and Bullough, *The Care of the Sick,* chaps. 7–10, addresses the national scene.

19. McCullough, "Nightingale Principles," 145.

20. Ibid., 148–68, 155.

21. Ibid., 158. There are a great many student tales in an occasional nursing student publication, *White Caps,* which is only sporadically maintained in the Montana State University Library archives. Also, the Great Falls students in 1917 compiled a scrapbook that reiterates many student experiences. In most respects the young women were like

other nursing students; see, e.g., Adelaide M. Nutting and Lavinia L. Dock, *A History of Nursing*, 4 vols. (New York: G. P. Putnam's Sons, 1907), esp. vols. 1 and 2.

22. McCullough, "Nightingale Principles," 158, cites an orientation pamphlet for prospective students printed in Helena in 1915 and distributed to newcomers. The curricular changes are covered by occasional publication of *Requirements and Curriculum for Schools of Nursing in Montana and Nurse Practice Law* (Helena: n.p.); the 1934 edition is a good summary of the period covered. In 1937 the National League of Nursing proposed what became standard revisions: *Curriculum Guide for Schools of Nursing*.

23. McCullough, "Nightingale Principles," 158.

24. Bullough and Bullough, *The Care of the Sick*, 165–71: "The predictions of increasing unemployment for nurses made by the Grading Committee turned out to be all too accurate. The depression that followed the stock market crash of 1929 created widespread unemployment throughout society and nurses were no exception." See also Louise Fitzpatrick, "Nurses in American History; Nursing and The Great Depression," *American Journal of Nursing* 75 (1975): 2188–90.

25. Sherrick et al., *Nursing in Montana*, 76–79; Isabel M. Stewart, *The Education of Nurses* (New York: Macmillan, 1943).

26. Sherrick et al., *Nursing in Montana*, 10: "Since the relation of economic and social change to the development of nursing is daily becoming more apparent, it is further suggested that consideration be given to representation from the fields of economics and sociology." Thirteen of the twenty-four Montana schools of nursing closed during the Depression.

27. Robert Rydell, Jeffrey J. Safford, and Pierce Mullen, *In the People's Interest: A Centennial History of Montana State University* (Bozeman: Montana State University, 1992), chaps. 8 and 9; Sherrick et al., *History of Montana State University School of Nursing*.

28. This topic is well represented in the literature from the national perspective, with clear resonance in Montana. See Bullough and Bullough, *The Care of the Sick*, 186–217. For anecdotal but insightful material, see Thelma M. Schorr and Anne Zimmerman, *Making Choices, Taking Chances: Nurse Leaders Tell Their Stories* (St. Louis: C. V. Mosby, 1988); of interest to a Nevada study is the account of Marlene F. Kramer on pp. 171–74. In Montana, small hospitals in particular have seen their nurses possessing higher degrees become increasingly independent. Biomedical technology is driving some changing perspectives even more radically than social mores or expectations might.

29. Dean of Science Division, Cotner correspondence, letter of May 26, 1947, Montana State University Archives, Sci I, folder 22, box N3, 569.

30. Mary Thompson Toy [nursing supervisor in Great Falls] to Dean Cotner, April 16, 1948, in Cotner correspondence.

31. Dean Cotner to R. K. Shiro [director of Great Falls Deaconess Hospital], October 22, 1948, in Cotner correspondence.

32. R. B. Richardson [president of the medical staff, Great Falls Deaconess] to Dean Cotner, December 20, 1948; and Miss Haza [outgoing director of nursing, Great Falls] to R. K. Shiro, June 8, 1950, both in Cotner correspondence.

33. Mary Anne Hugo [new director of nursing, Great Falls] to Anna Pearl Sherrick, March 8, 1950, Cotner correspondence.

34. Rev. E. L. Cooke [minister, First Methodist Church, Great Falls] to Dean Cotner October 7, 1950, both in Cotner correspondence.

35. J. Homer Magee [district supervisor of the Montana Conference of the Methodist church] to Dean Cotner, November 3, 1950, in Cotner correspondence.

36. Magee to Cotner, November 8, 1950, in Cotner correspondence.

37. Cotner to Mrs. Merriman, December 8, 1950, in Cotner correspondence.

38. Nena Neill Saunders, "Frontier Nursing: Nursing Practice in Medical Assistance Facilities Staffed by Physician Assistants" (master's thesis, Montana State University, 1992), 42; for other sources of personal stress, see 38–67.

8. Chinese Medicine on the "Gold Mountain": Tradition, Adaptation, and Change

This essay is largely based on fieldwork conducted in Boise, Idaho, and Seattle, Washington, between the years 1979 and 1985. My thanks to the Idaho and Washington Commissions for the Humanities for partially funding this research and to my co-worker Christopher Muench, who has generously shared with me his own insights regarding the Ah-fong materials over the years.

1. An introduction to the history of Chinese settlement of the United States is Douglas W. Lee, "The Advancing Chinese Frontier in America," in *Chinese Medicine on the Golden Mountain, an Interpretive Guide,* ed. Henry G. Schwarz (Bellingham, Wash.: n.p., 1984), 5–24.

2. I follow the convention of referring to "herbalists" and "herbal medicine," although strictly speaking, Chinese "herbal" medicine makes use of animal and mineral as well as plant drugs. Of 1,892 *materiae medicae* listed in the great sixteenth-century compendium *Pen-ts'ao kang-mu,* only 62 percent are from plants; 23.5 percent are from animals, and 14.5 percent are mineral.

3. That bone setting took place is evident from the number of recipes intended as supplementary herbal treatments for bone breaks in both the Seattle *Yao-fang* and the surviving Ah-fong materials. The practice is otherwise little documented. See, however, Christopher Muench, "One Hundred Years of Medicine, the Ah-fong Physicians of Idaho," in *Chinese Medicine,* ed. Schwarz, 64–65. Although moxacautery is not documented in written sources pertaining to the early Chinese pharmacies of the frontier West, the substantial quantities of prepared moxa surviving from the Ah-fong collection belonging to the Idaho Historical Society indicate that it was practiced; see ibid., 67–68.

4. Traditional dietary therapy is probably the form of traditional Chinese medicine most widely practiced within the family. According to the late Willard Chew, nearly every Chinese family in his time had one or more experts in dietary therapy who served as advisers to the rest. Willard himself was among them and is remembered as being particularly concerned about the color balance of foods served at banquets; sometimes foods had to be dyed with food coloring to make the rules work! The color of Chinese foods is important because it relates to the foods' healing or cooling qualities. Red foods such as red chilies are almost always considered heating, while green vegetables are generally regarded as cooling. If one has a condition caused by cold factors (e.g., some but

not all "colds"), one should eat heating foods; if one's system is overheated, cooling foods are called for. Since so many illnesses are due to poor nutrition, the system works well enough. See E. N. Anderson, "Why Is Humoral Medicine So Popular?" *Social Science and Medicine* 25 (1987): 331–37.

5. Most sources repress this aspect of Chinese healing, but among surviving materials from early Seattle pharmacies are several talismans. A talisman is usually a small piece of paper on which some special symbol is drawn that is placed in the room of the sick person to drive away evil influences. On being asked about such practices, Seattle's Hen Sen said that while he personally did not believe in the efficacy of talismans, he was willing to use them if his patient did.

6. The interpretation here follows closely that of Paul U. Unschuld in his *Medicine in China: A History of Ideas* (Berkeley: University of California Press, 1985); and, on the early history of Chinese acupuncture, Yamada Keiji, *Shinhatsugen Chūgoku kagakushi shiryō no kenkyū*, 2 vols. (Kyotō: Kyotō Daigaku Jinbun Kagaku Kenkyūjo, 1985). I am particularly grateful to Prof. Unschuld for our many discussions of Chinese medical theory and practice over the years and to Prof. Yamada for providing reprints of his important work.

7. The character for *doctor*, now written with an element meaning "bottle" (i.e., "drug") below it, was once written with the word separately used for male shaman in that position.

8. On China's herbal literature, see Paul U. Unschuld, *Medicine in China: A History of Pharmaceutics* (Berkeley: University of California Press, 1986).

9. Quotations from the *Yin-shan cheng-yao* (*szu-pu ts'ung-k'an hsü-pien*) are from Paul D. Buell and Eugene N. Anderson, *A Soup for the Qan: Chinese Dietary Medicine of the Mongol Era as Seen in Hu Szu-hui's Yin-shan cheng-yao* (London: Kegan Paul International, forthcoming, 1997).

10. See Unschuld, *Medicine in China: A History of Ideas*, 189ff. Unschuld recently published a complete translation of the works of an important medical thinker of the era; see Paul Unschuld, *Forgotten Traditions of Ancient Chinese Medicine, a Chinese View from the Eighteenth Century* (Brookline, Mass.: Paradigm Publications, 1990).

11. See Unschuld, *Medicine in China: A History of Ideas*, 212–13.

12. I am indebted to Christopher Muench for this insight.

13. See Paul D. Buell and Christopher Muench, "Chinese Medical Recipes from Frontier Seattle," *Annals of the Chinese Historical Society of the Pacific Northwest* 2 (1984): 100–43.

14. See Wolfram Eberhard, "Economic Activities of a Chinese Temple in California," in *Collected Papers*, vol. 1: *Settlement and Social Change in Asia* (Hong Kong: Hong Kong University Press, 1967), 264–78.

15. In the above recipes, a *ch'ien* is 3.12 grams, or 0.011 ounce, and is one-tenth of a *liang*. Sixteen *liang* make a *chin* (ca. 500 grams).

16. On the Ah-fong apothecary, see Paul Buell and Christopher Muench, "A Chinese Apothecary in Frontier Idaho," *Annals of the Chinese Historical Society of the Pacific Northwest* 1 (1983): 39–48; Christopher Muench, "Chinese Medicine in America, a Study in Adaptation," *Caduceus* 4 (1988): 5–35; and Muench, "One Hundred Years," 67.

17. See Unschuld, *Medicine in China: A History of Pharmaceutics,* 108ff.

18. See Buell and Muench, "Chinese Medical Recipes," 103.

19. Christopher Muench, personal communication. On the use of snakes and other reptiles in Chinese medicine, see Bernard E. Read, *Chinese Materia Medica,* vol. 7: *Dragons and Snakes* (Peiping: French Bookstore, 1934).

20. Christopher Muench, personal communication.

21. See Muench, "One Hundred Years," 67, 73, 76.

22. Ibid., 65.

23. Ibid., 68ff.; Muench, "Chinese Medicine in America," 16ff.

24. Jeffrey Barlow and Christine Richardson, *China Doctor of John Day* (Portland, Ore.: Binford & Mort, 1979).

25. I am indebted to Dr. Turner and her colleagues for sharing the results of their research with me.

26. This trend is touched on in passing in Paul Unschuld's *Die Praxis des traditionellen chinesischen Heilsystems,* Münchener Ostasiatische Studien 8 (Wiesbaden: Franz Steiner Verlag, 1973).

27. Personal communication.

28. This term is Hen Sen's.

Marie I. Boutté holds a Ph.D. in cultural anthropology and is an associate professor in the Department of Anthropology, University of Nevada, Reno. She has published widely in major journals in her field reflecting her research in medical anthropology on topics such as stigma and inherited diseases in the Azores Islands. In 1994 she began work on medical ethnographies in rural Nevada communities near the Nevada Test Site.

Paul D. Buell has a Ph.D. in history and an M.A. in Chinese. He is at home in fields as diverse as biomedical history, ethnobiology, the study of Central Asia, medieval Scandinavia, and the American West. He is the author or coauthor of four books and more than forty articles.

Alan Derickson is an associate professor of labor studies and history at Pennsylvania State University, University Park. He received his Ph.D. from the Department of the History of Health Sciences, University of California, San Francisco. His book *Workers' Health, Workers' Democracy: The Western Miners' Struggle, 1891–1925* (Cornell University Press) won the Philip Taft Labor History Award for 1988.

Diane D. Edwards is a doctoral candidate in the History of Science and Medicine, University of Wisconsin-Madison. She also has master's degrees in medical microbiology and mass communications and has been a laboratory researcher, a newspaper and magazine journalist, a freelance writer and textbook editor, a university lecturer and academic adviser, and an AIDS educator. She is now at Montana State University as a premed advisor while completing her Ph.D. on the history of Native American health care.

Victoria A. Harden is the historian for the National Institutes of Health and the director of the DeWitt Stetten Jr. Museum of Medical Research. In 1990 she published *Rocky Mountain Spotted Fever: History of a Twentieth-Century Disease* (Johns Hopkins University Press), and in 1995 she coedited *AIDS and the Public Debate: Historical and Contemporary Perspectives,* in addition to contributing a chapter on the NIH response to AIDS to that volume. Her interests focus on twentieth-century biomedical research, especially the history of infectious diseases and medical research instrumentation.

Martha L. Hildreth has a Ph.D. in history and is an associate professor of history at the University of Nevada, Reno. She is the author of *Doctors, Bureaucrats and Public Health in France, 1888–1902* (Garland, 1987). Her recent publications include articles on etiology and public health aspects of the 1918–19 influenza epidemic and on the construction of family-oriented private practice medicine in France.

Bruce T. Moran has a Ph.D. in history and is a professor of history at the University of Nevada, Reno. He is the author of numerous monographs and articles on Early Modern German science and medicine, including *The Alchemical World of the German Court* (Franz Steiner, 1991), *Chemical Pharmacy Enters the University: Johannes Hartmann and the Didactic Care of Chemiatria* (American Institute for the History of Pharmacy, 1991), and an edited volume, *Patronage and Institutions* (Boydell, 1991).

Pierce C. Mullen, a professor of history at the University of Montana, received his Ph.D. in the history of science and has since focused on nineteenth- and twentieth-century German developmental biology. He has published a history of the American Simmental Society and has written articles on Rocky Mountain spotted fever and the 1918–19 influenza epidemic in Montana.

Ronald L. Numbers is Hilldale and William Coleman Professor of the History of Science and Medicine at the University of Wisconsin-Madison. He is the author of numerous articles and fourteen books, among them *The Creationists* (Knopf, 1992). He has served on the councils of the American Association of the History of Medicine, the History of Science Society, and the American Society of Church History. Professor Numbers has recently been the editor of *ISIS,* the journal of the History of Science Society, and is currently working on a history of science in America for the Cambridge History of Science series.

Thomas J. Wolfe obtained a B.F.A. in theater from Boston University and then worked for a time as a stage manager and designer. He subsequently studied history at the University of Nevada and the history of science and medicine at the University of Wisconsin-Madison. He is currently writing his Ph.D. dissertation, "The Thomsonians: Medicine, Religion, and Popular Culture in Early Nineteenth-Century America."

INDEX

Page references to figures and illustrations are printed in bold type.

Ackerknecht, Erwin H., 7, 8
acquired immunodeficiency syndrome.
    See AIDS
acupuncture, 97, 99, 105
adaptation, medical, xix, 26, 90, 93–94,
    97–101, 104–9; and AIDS, 65–69; and
    germ theory, 59–65, 70–71. *See also*
    frameworks, intellectual
Ah-fong, C. K., 104–7
Ah-fong, Gerald, xvi, 59–71, 107
AIDS (acquired immunodeficiency syn-
    drome), xiv, 59, 65–69, **70**, **71**
Alaska, **12**, 13
Alberta, Canada, 15, 43, 45, 56
Albuquerque, New Mexico, 9
alchemist, Chinese, 96, 99, 104, 108. *See
    also* pharmacy
alcohol consumption, xv, 14, 22, 30, 53,
    106
Alcott, William, 22
alignment of heavenly bodies: as cause of
    disease, 60
Allegheny Mountains, 6
Allen, R. A., 48
allopathy, xviii
altitude therapy, 9
American Medical Association (AMA), 20,
    52

American Nurses' Association. *See* nurs-
    ing, associations
American Public Health Association
    (APHA), 72–74
American South, xv, 3, 4, 7–8, 16
analytical framework. *See* frameworks,
    intellectual
Anderson, John, 65
Anglicans. *See* Episcopalians
Annales school, 2
anorexia nervosa, xv
anthracosis, 81
anthrax, 64
anthropod-borne disease, 64–65, 72
anthropology, medical, xvii
antibiotics, 60, 108, 109
antimony, 26
Apaches, 44. *See also* Native Americans
Appalachian Mountains, 7
Ariss, E. Augusta, 85–87, 89
Arizona, 78, 79, 81
Arnold, David, xiv, xv
arsenic, 26, 106
Artemisia, 96
arthritis, 105, 106
Association of American Geographers, **14**
Atlanta, Idaho, 106
Atlantic Coastal Plain, 7

bacteria, 60, 61, 63

Baechler, Jean, 35–36; and classification of suicide motives, 36–38

Bahn, Anita, 73

Banks, Nathan, 65

Baptists, 20–21

bayberry bark, 26

behaviors: as cause of disease, 14, 71. *See also* occupational disease

Bennett, John Cook, 25, 27

Benton, Mehitabel, 19

Betts, William W., 75, 76

biopathology, xv, xvi, 60–69, 73–76

birthrates, 55

Bitterroot Valley, Montana, 8, 62, 65

Blackfeet Agency (Montana), xviii; conditions at, 43–58

Blackfoot Confederacy, 43–58. *See also* Native Americans

blindness, 46

Bloods (tribe), 45. *See also* Native Americans

boarding schools, 45, **47,** 50

Board of Indian Commissioners. *See* Blackfeet Agency

boards of health, 25, 62, 64, 78

Boise, Idaho, 102, 104, 106, 107

bone setting, 96

Boutté, Marie I., xvii, 29–42

Braudel, Fernand, 2

Brother Van. *See* Orsdel, W. W. van

Browning, Montana, 46

Buddhism, 99

Buell, Paul D., xviii, 95–109

Buley, R. Carlyle, 4

Bureau of Indian Affairs (BIA), xiv, 56, 58

Bureau of Land Management, xiv, 33–34

Bureau of Mines (BOM), 80, 81

Butte, Montana, 77, 80

Butte Anti-Tuberculosis Society, 80

byssinosis, 81

caffeine, 22

California, 62, 67

calomel (mercurial compound), 23

Campbell, Fred, 48, 50, 51, 54

Campbellite Disciples of Christ, 21

Canada, **10,** 15, 57–58; medical school locations in, **10**

cancer, 66–68, 108

canker, 26

Cannon, Dr., 26

Cascade Mountains, xiii, 62

Catholic hospitals, 17, 85, 88–89

Centers for Disease Control (CDC), 30–32, 67

chi, 103

ch'i, 98–100

childbirth, 20, 55

Chin Hen Sen. *See* Hen Sen (Chin)

Chinese medicine, xiii, xviii, 95–109

Ch'in Shih-huang-ti, 95

chiropractic, 20

chloroform, 26

cholera, xiv, 64, 72; and waterborne disease, 62

The Cholera Years (Rosenberg), 20

"chosen of Nauvoo," 27

Chowning, Wilson M., 62, 63, 65

Church of Jesus Christ of Latter-day Saints. *See* Mormons

cigarette smoking, 14

class, 2–4, 97

Clemens, Samuel (Mark Twain), 8

climate, 5, 8–9, 46, 74

climatotherapy. *See* altitude therapy

collectivistic cultures, 40

Colorado, 8, 11, 15, 61, 74, 79, 82; and AIDS, 67

Colorado Medicine. See Rocky Mountain Medical Journal

Committee on the Costs of Medical Care. *See* health care, planners

Comstock mines, 73; and suicide, 29

concept of ideal types (Weber), 36

Congregationalists, 20–21

construct, intellectual. *See* frameworks, intellectual

consumption. *See* tuberculosis

continued fever. *See* typhus

contract physicians, 16, 44

correspondence theory, 100, 101, 104

Cotner, Frank B., 90–92

Council of Health, 26

Crabbe, Theodore, 55

Creviston, Warren R., 49

Cultural Regions of the United States
(Gastil), 2

cultural response, 3, 14, 40; to suicide,
xvii, 31, 35–42. *See also* frameworks,
intellectual; regionalism; Thomsonianism

Cut Bank, Montana, **47,** 52

cytokines, 60

Deaconess: hospitals, 51, 85, 87, 90, 91;
movement, xviii, 82–94

death: infant, 52, 56; rate, 46, 52, 55–57, 58;
by suicide, xv, xvii, 29, 32, 34–42

DeLaMar: Joseph R., 74; Nevada Gold
Mining Company, 74; town of, in
Nevada, 74–76

demon possession, 97–98, 109

dental disease, 49

Denver and Gross College of Medicine
(Colorado), 11

Department of Health, Education, and
Welfare (HEW), 43–44, 56

Department of the Interior, xviii, 43–46,
48–53, 56, 58

De Quille, Dan, 73

Derickson, Alan, xvii, xviii, 72–81

Dermacentor andersoni, 61, 65

Dermacentor venustus, 65

Deseret News, 25

de Smet, Father, 82

diarrhea, 57

dietary manual, Chinese, 99, 102–3, 105,
109

dietary therapy, 6, 96. *See also* dietary
manual, Chinese; nutrition

disease, ix, xix; anthropod-borne, 64–65;

causes of, xv, xvi, 14, 60–62, 71, 97–100;
identifying new, ix, 59–71; of nature,
60–61; theory of, xiv–xv, xvi, 6, 59, 68;
tick-borne, 8, 63, 65; waterborne, 62.
See also frameworks, intellectual

disease determinants: environment, 60–
61, 72; geological, 6; meterological, 6;
occupational, xvii, 14, 33–35, 71, 72–81,
104, 106; political, 43–58, 72; social,
xiii, xviii, 6, 14, 18–42, 67–68, 70, 72

divorce, 14, 30

DNA (deoxyribonucleic acid), 66

doctor-pharmacist, 96

*Doctors of Medicine in New Mexico: A
History of Health and Medical Practice,
1886–1986* (Spidel), **9**

Doctrine and Covenants. *See* Mormons

Drake, Daniel, 5–7

Duesberg, Peter, 69

Duncan, Dayton, 39–40

dust disease. *See* miners' consumption

dynamite, 73, 77

dysentery, leaking, 99

Eberhard, Wolfram, 102

economy: disease and, xiii, 44, 48–52, 67,
72; suicide and, xvii, 32–35, 41–42

education, medical. *See* schools

Edwards, Diane D., xvii, 43–58

Ellis, John H., 8

Ely, Nevada, xvii, 31, 32, 40; suicide in,
xvii, 31–42

empiricist view of disease, xv. *See also*
frameworks, intellectual

Encyclopedia of Southern Culture, 3

Engineering and Mining Journal, 74

environment: as disease determinant, xvi,
7, 60–61, 72

epidemic, xvii, 57, 72–74; AIDS, 67; silicosis, 72–81

epidemiology, xvi, 6–7, 59–71, 72–81; suicide and, 29–42

Epidemiology: Principles and Methods
(MacMahon and Pugh), 73

Episcopalians, 20–21

Epworth League Methodist Episcopal Church, 88

erysipelas, 53

ether, 26

Etheridge, Elizabeth W., 8

Ettling, John, 7, 8

faith healing, 22–23, 25, 96

falciparum malaria, 7

family right (Thomsonian), 19, 23

Farmer, David, 76

female complaints, 106

feng, 97

fever, mountain. *See* Rocky Mountain spotted fever

field matrons, 46, 49, 50, 54. *See also* nursing

Fife, Austin, 26

Firth, Raymond, 42

Flexner, Abraham, **10**, 11

Fliedner: nursing model, 94; Theodore, 83–84

flu. *See* influenza

Foard, Fred T., 58

Forest Service, 33

Fox, Daniel M., 13

Fox, L. Webster, 50–51

foxtail millet, 99, 100

frameworks: AIDS, 65–71; Chinese, 97–101, 104, 108; germ theory, xv, xvi, 5, 59–60, 63, 66, 68, 70; intellectual, for understanding disease, xv, xvi, xvii, 19, 59–71; Koch's postulates, 64, 68, 69, 125n21; limits of, 70; predictive possibilities, 68; Rocky Mountain spotted fever, 60–65

Framing Disease: Studies in Cultural History (Rosenberg and Golden), xv

Fred Victor Rescue Mission, 85

free silica, 72, 75; and permissible exposure limit, 80

Friendly Botanic Society, 19, 20

From Saddlebags to Scanners: The First 100 Years of Medicine in Washington State (Rockafellar and Haviland), **12**

Fuchs, Victor R., 13

Fuller, Blanch, 51

Gallo, Robert C., 68, 69

gangrene, 23

Gastil, Raymond D., 2

General Education Board, 11

geography, xiii, xvi, xvii, 27, 59, 61, 66–67, 70–71; suicide and, xvii, 40. *See also* specificity, doctrine of

germ theory, 5, 59, 60, 63, 66, 68, 70–71

Glacier National Park, 45, 57

Goldfield, Nevada, 41

Goldman, Marion, 29

"Gold Mountain," xiii, xviii, 95–109

gonorrhea, 104; cure for, 102–3

gout, 106

Government Accounting Office, 52

Graham, Sylvester, 22

Great Basin, xiii

Great Basin National Park, 33

Great Falls, Montana, 51

Great Falls Deaconess Hospital, 85, 87, 90

Green River, 62

GRID (gay-related immune disorder), 66. *See also* AIDS

Grollman, Earl, 30

Gros Ventres, 45. *See also* Native Americans

group practice, 16

Guelph General Hospital Nurses' Training School, 85

hangover remedy, 102–3

Harden, Victoria A., xv, xvi, 8, 59–71

Harrington, Daniel, 80

Harvard University Medical School, 64

Haviland, James W., **12**

healing, faith, 22–23, 25, 96

health care: planners, 13; system (defined), xiv

health needs: of miners, 72–81; of Mor-

mons, 18–28; of reservation tribes, 43–58; rural, 39, 42
Helena, Montana, 82
henbane, 26
Hen Sen (Chin), 101, 104, 105, 106, 107
herbal medicine, 18–20, 25–27; Chinese, xix, 96, 97, 98, 99–100, 102–5, 107–8. *See also* Chinese medicine; Thomsonianism
Higham, John, 2
Hill, J. J., 85
Hippocrates, 3
histocompatibility complexes, 60
HIV (human immunodeficiency virus). *See* AIDS
homeopathy, 20, 53. *See also* herbal medicine
Hong Kong, 108
hookworm, 7, 8
hospitals, xix, 17, 49, 51, 52, 55, 84–86, 88–89
host immune defenses, 59, 66. *See also* AIDS
Hotchkiss, Samuel, 79
housefly, 63
human behavior: as a cause of disease, xvi. *See also* alcohol consumption; dietary therapy; occupation; smoking
human-T-cell lymphotropic virus III (HTLV-III), 69. *See also* AIDS
Humphreys, Margaret, 8
Hu Szu-hui, 109
hydrographical map, 6
hydropathy, 20
Hygienic Laboratory, 63

Idaho, xiv, xix, 12–16, 51, 61
illness: suicide and, 35
immigration patterns, xiii, xiv, xviii, 18, 30, 76, 109
immune disease, 59, 60, 66, 70. *See also* AIDS
impotency, 105
Independence Rock, 62

India: medical system borrowed from, 99
Indians. *See* Native Americans
Indian Service, 44, 45, 48–50, 55, 56; hospitals, 52
Indian tobacco (*Lobelia inflata*): medicinal properties of, 19. *See also* tobacco
individualistic cultures, 40
industrial disease, 74, 106. *See also* occupational disease
infantile diarrhea, 57
infant mortality, 49, 52, 56
infection, 64; opportunistic, 66, 67
influenza, 54, 87
Ing Hay, 107
Insects and Disease (Doane), 63
Institute for Government Research, 48
Institut Pasteur (Paris), 68, 69
insurance, medical, 4, 89
intermittent fever. *See* malaria
International Association for Suicide Prevention, 38
International Commission on Zoological Nomenclature, 65
Islamic medicine, 103, 109
isolation, xiii, xiv, xviii, 16, 27, 30, 40, 42, 56, 74

John Day, Oregon, 40, 102, 107
Journal of American History, 3
Journal of the American Medical Association, 76

Kaiserwerth program, 84
Karposi's sarcoma, 66. *See also* AIDS
Kennecott Copper Company, 33
Kindall, Cleve E., 81
Kirtland, Ohio, 21, 24
Koch, Robert, 5, 64
Koch's postulates, 64, 68–69, 125n21. *See also* frameworks, intellectual
Kunitz, Stephen, 57, 58

LaFarge, Oliver, 58
Lake Tahoe, 8

Lamb, Miss, 87
Lanza, Anthony J., 79, 80
Lapwai Sanatorium (Idaho), 51
Last Chance Gulch, Helena, Montana, 82
Las Vegas, Nevada, 13, 32
laughing gas, 26
LAV (lymphadenophy-associated virus),
    69. *See also* AIDS
laws: licensing, 20, 107; mining, 78, 81; re-
    stricting dispensing of medical sub-
    stances, 25–26
"lazy diseases," 7
Leadville, Colorado, 74, 82
leukemia, 68
Life magazine, 32, 40
Lincoln County, Nevada, 74
"The Loneliest Road in America," 32, **33**,
    40
Long, Kathleen Ann, 39–42
Lowney, John, 77
lung disease. *See* pneumoconiosis; pneu-
    monia; silicosis; tuberculosis
Lung On, 107
lymphatic system, 66

MacMahon, Brian, 73
Magee, J. Homer, 92, 93
magic, 96
Magma Nevada Mining Company, 34
malaria, 6–8, 63
Malaria in the Upper Mississippi Valley
    (Ackerknecht), 8
Mandans, 44. *See also* Native Americans
marriage, plural, 22, 26, 27
Marysville, California, 102
Mausner, Judith, 73
Maxey, Edward E., 61
McGill, Nevada, 32
McKeown, Thomas, xv
measles, 56
Medical Advocate (Thomsonian journal),
    19
medical associations. *See* medical societies

medical education. *See* medical schools;
    schools
*Medical Education in the United States
    and Canada: A Report to the Carnegie
    Foundation for the Advancement of
    Teaching* (Flexner), 10
medical facilities, 8–13, 16, 45–55
medical history, xiv, xv, xix; Chinese, 95–
    102, 106–9; miners', 72–81; nursing,
    82–94; significance of regions in, 1–17;
    of suicide, 29–42; of Thomsonian
    movement, 18–28
medical insurance, 4, 89
medical literature: Chinese, 98–106, 109
medical practice, xiv, xix; Chinese, 95–
    109; contract physicians, 16, 44; group,
    16; Mormon, 17, 18–20, 22, 23, 25–26;
    nursing, 39, 90–91; small town, xiv,
    xix, 39, 42
medical reform, 13, 20–23
medical regionalism, xv, 1–17
medical schools, xiv, 4, 9–13; Chicago
    Homeopathic College, 53; Denver and
    Gross College of Medicine, 11; Har-
    vard University Medical School, 64;
    Marquette University, 53; Stanford
    University School of Medicine, 51;
    University of Colorado School of
    Medicine, 11; University of Utah,
    11; University of Washington, 13;
    Western University of Canada, 53
Medical Sentinel, 16
medical societies, 15, 16, 20, 26, 52, 86
medical theory: Chinese, 95–109; germ, 5,
    59, 60, 63, 66, 68, 70. *See also* frame-
    works, intellectual
medical tinctures (Chinese), 105
medicinal plants: Chinese, 99–106; and
    Native American tradition, 43; and
    Thomsonianism, 18–20
medicine, and religion, xviii, 2, 82–89,
    99, 106. *See also* Chinese medicine,
    medicinal plants, Thomsonianism

*The Mediterranean and the Mediterra-
nean World in the Age of Philip II*
(Braudel), 2
Meeks, Priddy, 26, 28
Meinig, D. W., 14
meningitis, 48
Mennonites, 84
mercury, 23, 26, 104–6
Merriman, Marjorie, 92, 93
Merrit, E. B., 51
Methodist City, Home, and Foreign Mis-
sions Office, 85
Methodists, xviii, 20, 21, 23, 88, 92; Dea-
coness movement, 82–94; Mormons
and, 24
Meyer, Lucy Rider, 85
miasmas: as cause of disease, 62
*The Midwest Pioneer: His Ills, Cures and
Doctors* (Pickard and Buley), 4
midwives, 20, 26, 88
*Miles from Nowhere: Tales from America's
Contemporary Frontier* (Duncan),
39–40
Miller, M. A., 54
miners' consumption, xvii, 72–81. *See also*
silicosis
Mine Safety and Health Administration,
80
mining, xiii, xvii, 33–34, 72–81, 104
Minnesota nursing school model, 89
Mintzer, O. W., 85
missionaries, 44, 83; medicine and, 16–17
Mississippi Valley area, 8
Mongolian medicine, 109
Montagnier, Luc, 68–69
Montana, xiv, xvii, xviii, 8, 12, 13, 39, 77,
82; nursing in, 83, 84–94. *See also*
Blackfeet Agency
Montana Deaconess Hospital, 51, 85, 91
Montana Methodist Mission, 85
Montana State Association of Graduate
Nurses. *See* nursing, associations
Montana State Board of Health, 62, 64

Montana State College (MSC) nursing
program. *See* nursing, schools
Montana State Hospital for the Feeble
Minded, 51
Montana Tuberculosis Association, 54
moral defect: as cause of disease, 60
"The Mormon Culture Region: Strategies and Patterns in the Geography
of the American West, 1847–1964"
(Meinig), **14**
Mormons, xiii, xvi, xviii, 14, 18–28; Doctrine and Covenants, 22; as exception
to other immigration patterns, xiv;
and polygamy, 22, 26, 27; and Thomsonianism, 18–28; and "Word of Wisdom," 22
Morse, William, 26
mortality. *See* death
mosquito, 63
mountain fever. *See* Rocky Mountain
spotted fever
mountain sickness. *See* Rocky Mountain
spotted fever
mountain typhus. *See* Rocky Mountain
spotted fever
moxacautery, 96, 98
Moyer, Charles, 79
Mullen, Pierce C., xviii, 82–94
Muslim medicine, 103, 109

Nash, Roy, 49
National Cancer Institute, 68
National Institutes of Health (NIH), 66, 68
nationalism: influence of, on acceptance
of Thomsonianism, 20
National Research Council, 67
National Tuberculosis Association, 48
"nation of sections," 1
Native Americans, xiii, xvii, 29, 41, 43–58;
health of, 43–58; life expectancy of,
52; and medical practices, xix; on
the reservation, xviii, 43–58; suicide
and, 41

naturalism: influence of, on acceptance of Thomsonianism, 20

Nature magazine, 69

Nauvoo, Illinois, 22, 25

Nauvoo Legion, 24

Navajos, 57. *See also* Native Americans

Nazarene, 88

necessity argument, 64, 69

Neoconfucianism, 99. *See also* frameworks, intellectual

neurasthenia, xv

Nevada, xiv, 13–15, 62, 72, 76, 79; suicide in, 29–42

Nevada Board of Health, 78

Nevada Vital Statistics Report, 30, 32, 34

New Deal health policy, 89

A New Guide to Health (Thomson), 19, 26

New Mexico, xiv, 9, 15

Newton, Elsie, 46

Nightingale: Florence, 84; nursing model, 83, 94; Pledge, 86

nightshade, 26

night sweats, 76

nomenclature, disease, 65

North Dakota, 44

Northern Montana Mission, 85

Numbers, Ronald L., xv, xvi, xix, 1–17

nurse practitioners, 88, 93

nursing, xviii, 50, 55, 82–94; apprenticeship, 87–93; associations, 86; and Blackfeet Agency, 49; field matrons, 46, 49, 50, 54; history of, xviii, 82; practices and standards, 39, 90, 91; practitioners of, 88, 93; schools, 82, 85, 87–94

nutrition, xv, 44, 46, 47, 57, 138n4. *See also* dietary manual, Chinese; dietary therapy

Oatman, Arizona, 81

obstetrics, 20, 26, 88

occupation: suicide and, xvii, 33–35

occupational disease, xv, xvii, 14, 72–81, 104, 106

Old, H. Norman, 58

On Airs, Waters, and Places (Hippocrates), 3–4

Ontario, Canada, 82

opium, 26

Oregon, 15, 16, 40, 61–62, 102, 107

Orsdel, W. W. van (Brother Van), 85, 87

Orthopedic Commission, 87

osteopathy, 20

Pacific Medical Record, 16

Palmyra, New York, 21

paradigms: for understanding disease, 60. *See also* frameworks, intellectual

Parkinson's disease, 108

Pasteur, Louis, 5

patterns of disease. *See* frameworks, intellectual

Patterson, K. David, 7

pediatrics, 88

pellagra, 7, 8

pen-ts'ao, 98–100, 104

pharmacy, xviii, 4, 25–26, 96, 98–109

philosophy, medical: Chinese, 98–100. *See also* frameworks, intellectual

Phipps Institute (Philadelphia), 52

physicians, 53–54; roles and responsibilities of, xix; rural, xiv, xix; women, 83, 94. *See also* medical schools

physiographic regions, 2

The Physiography of the United States (Powell), 2

Pickard, Madge E., 4

Piegans (tribe), 45. *See also* Native Americans

Pike's Peak (Colorado), 8

Piroplasma hominis, 63

place: concept of, xvi, 4, 27, 59, 61, 70, 71. *See also* regionalism

pneumoconiosis, xvii, 72, 73, 75, 77, 80; dry drilling and, xvii, 78, 81

pneumonia, 57

pneumothorax procedure, 51

"poison doctor," 26

poison (strong medicinal effect), 100

polygamy, 22, 26, 27

Poplar River Indians, 54. *See also* Native Americans

Poplin, Missouri, 79

Powell, John Wesley, 1, **2**, 29

Presbyterians, 20–21

prescriptions, 19, 26; formulas (Chinese), 108; individualistic, 60

prevention: disease, 46; by how the disease is constructed, 68

Primitive Physic (Wesley), 23

prison, 33, 41

"Problems in American History" (Powell), 1

process of disease. *See* biopathology

profile, suicide risk, 31

prostitution, 29, 30, 106

Protestant, 87

protozoa, 60, 63

public health, xvi, 4, 7, 13, 43. *See also* American Public Health Association (APHA); Public Health Service, U.S.

Public Health and Marine Hospital Service, U.S., 63, 65, 79

Public Health Service, U.S. (PHS), 13, 46, 52, 56, 79–81

Pugh, Thomas F., 73

purpura, palpable, 61

race, 2–4

ranching, xiii, xvii

rattlesnake wine, 105

Red Cross, 87

regionalism, xiii, xiv–xvi, xviii, 1–17; as analytical framework for studying disease, xv, 79–81; hierarchical, xvi; identity and, xv, xvi, 4; medical, xv, xix, 3–17

Regional Medical Program (RMP), 13

regions, xv, xvi, 1–17; epidemiological, 7, 60–70, 72–81; suicide and, 29–42

religion, xviii, 2, 18–28, 56, 58, 99, 106; Baptist, 20, 21; Catholic, 17, 88–89;

Congregationalist, 20, 21; Methodist, xviii, 20, 21, 23, 24, 88, 92; Methodist Deaconess movement, 82–89; missionaries, 16–17, 44, 82–89; Mormon, xiii, xvi, xviii, 14, 18–28; Protestant, 87; Thomsonianism and, 18–28

Reno, Nevada, 13, 32

Reno Gazette-Journal, 34

republicanism: influence of, on acceptance of Thomsonianism, 20

research opportunities, xix, 13, 34, 39, 41–42, 57

reservations. *See* Native Americans

respiratory disease, occupational, 72–81

retrovirus, 65–66, 68–69. *See also* AIDS

rheumatism, 105

Richards, Levi and Willard, 24, 26

Richardson, R. B., 91

Ricketts, Howard Taylor, 63, 64, 69

rickettsiae, 8, 61, 63, 64, 69, 70

Riggin, R. A., 85

risk, suicide and, 42; RNA (ribonucleic acid), 65–66

Rockafellar, Nancy, **12**

Rocky Mountain Medical Association, 15

Rocky Mountain Medical Journal, xvi, 15

Rocky Mountain spotted fever, xvi, 8, 59–66, 69, 70–71

Rocky Mountain wood tick, 61, 65

Rogers, Frank B., 9

Roosevelt, Franklin D., 51

Root-Bernstein, Robert, 69

Rosenberg, Charles, xv, 20, 72

Rosin, Clifton, 48, 53

Roughing It (Mark Twain), 8

Ruth, Nevada, 32

Ruxton, George Frederick, 8

Ryan, Edward, 78

Salt Lake City, Utah, 11, 25, 32

Samek, Hana, 58

Sampson, Avard, 25

sanatoria, xix, 9, 55; tuberculosis, 51, 52

sanitation, lack of, 46, 57

Savitt, Todd, xv

Sayers, Royd, 80

schools: boarding, 45, **47,** 50; Canadian medical, 10; nursing, 82, 85, 87–94. *See also* medical schools

Schrader, Herman F., 48, 51–52

Science magazine, 69

scientific construction, xv, 57, 59–71; of AIDS, 65–66; new diseases and, 70–71; of Rocky Mountain spotted fever, 59, 68–71. *See also* frameworks, intellectual; germ theory; Koch's postulates

Scott, Hugh, 48

Seattle, Washington, 102

secularization: influence of, on nursing, 93

shamanic intervention, 96, 97, 100

Sharon, Vermont, 21

Sherrick, Anna Pearl, 90, 91–92

Shiro, C. K., 91

Shoshone: suicide and, 41. *See also* Native Americans

silicosis, xvii, 72–81

silico-tuberculosis, 76

Sills, J. C., 53

sisterhoods, nursing, 82

Sisters of Charity of Leavenworth, 82

situational association, xvi; vs. causative agent, 71

smallpox, 44, 46, 48, 57

Smith, Alvin, 22–23

Smith, Joseph, Jr., 21–24, 28; Sr., 21

smoking, 22

Snake River valley, 61

social constructionist view of disease, xv, 59–60, 68, 70

societies. *See* medical societies

South Africa: missionary to, 88; pneumoconiosis in, 77

South Dakota, 44

Southern Paiute: suicide among, 29. *See also* Native Americans

specificity, doctrine of, 4–6, 11. *See also* regionalism

Spidel, Jake W., Jr., 9

spotted fever. *See* Rocky Mountain spotted fever

St. George, Utah, 76

standing churches, 21

Stanford University School of Medicine, 51

starvation, 44, 46

State and Provincial Health Authorities of North America, 52

Stauffer, Dr., 53

"steam doctors," 19

Stiles, Charles Wardell, 63, 65

Stone, Forrest, 51, 55

studies, of disease, xv, 59–81. *See also* epidemiology

suicide, xvii, 29–42; cultural context of, xvii, 31, 35–42; demographics of, 34–35; methods of, 35; motives for, 35–42; rates, 29, 32, 34–35; risk factors, 29–31, 35–41; age groups, 34

Sweetwater River, 62

Systematic Treatise, Historical, Etiological, and Practical, on the Principal Diseases of the Interior Valley of North America (Drake), 5–6

Taft, William H., 50

Taiwan, 108

T'ang-pen chu, 100

T'ang-yeh pen-ts'ao (Wang Hao-ku), 104

Tao, 106

Taoist physiological alchemy, 99

tarsectomy, radical, 50

Texas, 67

Texas cattle fever, 65

theoretical framework for understanding disease. *See* frameworks, intellectual

theory: vs. practice, 101

theory of disease. *See* frameworks, intellectual

therapeutic locale, xix, 8–9. *See also* regionalism

The Therapeutic Perspective (Warner), 4
Thomson, John, 26
Thomson, Samuel, 18–21, 26, 28
Thomsonianism, xviii, 18–28, 43
tick-borne disease, 8, 63, 65
tinctures, medical, 102–3, 105
tobacco, 22
Tonopah, Nevada, 78, 81
Tonopah Miners' Union, 79
Townsend, James G., 52
trachoma, 46, 48–51; and radical tarsectomy, 50
trail typhus. *See* Rocky Mountain spotted fever
transient population, xiii, 30
transitional phases, five, 98, 99
tuberculosis (consumption), xvi, 8, 9, 48, 49, 56, 76; associations, 48, 54, 80; death rate, 52, 57, 58; pneumothorax procedure, 51; rate, 46, 50; sanatoria, 52; tubercule bacillus and, 64. *See also* altitude therapy
Turner, Frederick Jackson, xix, 93
Turner, Nancy, 107
typhoid fever, 63; and waterborne disease, 62
typhus, 6, 63

understandings of disease: by lay community, xvi. *See also* frameworks, intellectual
unemployment: suicide and, 34
union, 76, 77, 79, 92
Unitarian Universalist Association, 30
United States Botanic Convention, first, 20
universalism, scientific, xvi, 4
Universalists, 21
University of Colorado School of Medicine (Boulder), 11
University of Iowa, 12
University of Utah, 11, 13
University of Washington School of Medicine Primary Care Teaching Program (WAMI), 11–13
Utah, xiv, 11, 13–16, 62, 76

Vancouver, British Columbia, 102
venereal disease, 49, 104, 106. *See also* gonorrhea
virus, 60, 61, 66

Warner, John Harley, xv, 4–5
Wasatch Mountains, xiii
Wasatch Oasis, 14
Washington, 12, 16, 62
wasting, 66
Weber's concept of ideal types (suicide), 36
Weinert, Clarann, 39–42
Wesley, John, 23
West, Margaret Cooper, 25
Western Federation of Miners (WFM), xvii, 76, 77
Western Interstate Commission for Higher Education, 12
Western Journal of Medicine, 15
Western Medical Times, 16
Western Shoshone: and suicide, 41. *See also* Native Americans
Wheeler, Burton K., 49
White Cross Day, 88
"white father medicine." *See* Native Americans, health of
White Pine: County, Nevada, 31, 40; Power Project, 33; suicide in, 32
white plague. *See* tuberculosis
Williams, Frederick Granger, 23, 24
Wilson, Horace, 54
Wilson, Louis B., 62, 63, 65
Wing Luke Asian Museum, 104
Wolbach, Simeon Burt, 64
Wolfe, Thomas J., xviii, 18–28
women, 20, 83, 94, 106
Wood, Marshall W., 61
workers' compensation, 79

wounds, 104
Wyoming, xiv, 13, 15, 16, 62

Yao-fang, 102–5
Yellow Emperor's Inner Classic, 98, 99
yellow fever, 6–8, 65
yin and *yang,* 98, 99

Yin-shan cheng-yao (Chinese dietary
    manual), 99, 102–3, 105, 109
Young, Brigham, 22, 24
youth suicide, 34

Zanjani, Sally, 29